Eat,
Guilt,
Repent,
Repeat

Eat, Guilt, Repent, Repeat

Break the cycle!
Love your body, your food and your life!

Brenda J. Bentley
Cognitive Hypnotherapist and
Certified Intuitive Eating Counselor

Published By UnlimitedVision 12/04/2012

Notice: The information in this book is intended as a reference volume only. Any decisions you make about your lifestyle are your own and you remain wholly responsible for any decisions and actions you take. The information provided in this book is not a substitute for proper medical advice. If in doubt, please contact your doctor.

ISBN: 978-1-48125-325-3 (sc)

ISBN: 978-1-61979-339-6 (e)

This book is printed on acid-free paper.

Contents

This book is dedicated to all my clients who I have taught and who have taught me too.

You are an inspiration.

Foreword

Every once in a while, we are blessed with a book which seemingly appears out of nowhere. We cannot explain its reasons for arriving in our hands. It may be that we have picked it up at a bookstore, downloaded it on to our Kindle/iPad or perhaps have been gifted it. The reason does not matter as to how it is has been delivered to us.

You can trust that this book has been sent to you from a higher source, for your soul's expansion and this is something to really rejoice in. You may have been asking or perhaps praying for answers to your deep inner soul's longings, particularly related to weight issues. I'm pretty sure that the answer to many of your questions can be found here, in this book. It is designed to work with you on a mind, body & soul level. You will be working in partnership with the book and it will become a friend and support system to you if you choose.

If you are prepared to really stretch yourself, and are ready to allow some of these incredible changes to happen in your life right now, you will find that Brenda easily guides you throughout the book, in easy practical ways and I'm sure you will never look back! There are many incredible gems of wisdom in this book. It will be a book which can act as a guide, perhaps even as a friend, which you may like to refer to frequently, and it is timeless.

Brenda actively encourages taking responsibility for your own actions, and this book will help you to gently but powerfully do so. I personally believe we are presented with just the right tool at just the right time. Brenda has easily and effortlessly captured and explained many of the different facets of our human aspects & behavioural traits, which, we sometimes cannot understand. She helps explain different reasons for our reactions and actively gives us, the reader, wonderful simple steps to take which will create powerful results.

This is not just a book about weight loss, it is designed to help give you a clearer, broader & deeper understanding of what it really means to be at a place of peace within yourself, and which ultimately then helps to create the desired results.

This book which Brenda has so beautifully carved out, will take you on a journey, on a mind, body and soul level. It will leave you with a sense of awe and wonder. A deep realization that, you can indeed change anything you desire to change in your life. It brings a refreshing sense of freedom, lightness and wellbeing.

Brenda has expressed this wonderfully through a combination of her own experiences in life, and also through her clients' experiences & stories too. It's easy to relate to and is very practical. If you allow it, this book can be a lifelong friend and tool, used to guide you at any time, and it can and will help you change your life for the better.

Jolene Setterfield, June 2012
Intuitive Mentor, TV Personality & Author www.jolene.com

Introduction

This book was always going to be written, but it wasn't going to be about this. I had started out with the idea of bringing together all the written resources, homework and exercises I share with clients to support them outside of the therapy room. With my intention in mind, starting out and going with the flow of what life brought to me, it was clear this subject matter served the best purpose of my intention. It made sense, as most of my clients come to me for weight loss.

In my private practice as a cognitive hypnotherapist and integrative psychotherapist (which is a fancy term for a 'Jill of All Therapies' that has a lot of tools in her toolbox) my clients are looking for a quick fix. When I started out helping clients I thought that was my purpose. I had studied the 'Brief Therapy' model as outlined by Professor Rubin Battino and believed that everyone could benefit from some therapy, but that most of us don't need very much. I also found myself keen to focus on solutions instead of problems.

This approach was born out of my own journey where I've had my fair share of therapy to overcome my personal difficulties. Most of the therapy I undertook was because I needed help to resolve difficult past experiences from my childhood which continued to affect my present. These experiences gave me good insight into different therapeutic approaches that either worked or didn't work for me. It also refined a lifetime interest in psychology as a practical application instead of all the theory I learned in college.

The reality is that change is a process and there is no quick-fix to a long-term solution. This doesn't mean that you cannot have significant positive change in a short period of time. What I have learned is that there is no magic wand, magic words or magical treatment that will bring my clients what they want: to be fixed in under an hour.

In my practice, I use hypnotherapy as a tool to work with the unconscious learned behavior patterns. There are still misconceptions about what hypnotherapy is, and how it's touted as a mind-control tool, where the client surrenders their will over to the hypnotist who impregnates their mind with consensually agreed suggestions to change their problem behaviors. On one level, yes, willingness is key to change. You must be willing to change and consent to this in order to make change happen. This takes out the mind-control part of this misconception as you cannot control someone's mind who is giving you permission to do so! Still, there are many therapists that want to have the position whereby the power lies within them to change the client. I couldn't disagree more earnestly.

There is a Chinese proverb that says: "If you give a man a fish, you feed him for a day. If you teach a man to fish, you feed him for a lifetime."

And it was Karl Marx who said: "Sell a man a fish, he eats for a day, teach a man how to fish, you ruin a wonderful business opportunity."

So we see there was a mismatch of what clients wanted (a quick-fix) and what I was delivering (empowerment). Most clients come to me seeking to lose weight. What they learn is weight gain is often a symptom of something else. It's the result of an underlying poor relationship with food or with themselves. If it was true that weight is strictly a physical / biological result of the client's eating behaviors then diets would work.

Truth is that diets only work short-term. As you can appreciate, you can change something physically, but until you change the whole person including the emotional, psychological and spiritual, you are only applying a quick-fix for a short-term solution which will fade as soon as you stop doing it.

What you will find in the pages of this book and in the companion workbook/audio toolkit are the principles, lessons, strategies, tools and empowerment to make change to the WHOLE—the physical, mental, emotional, psychological and spiritual for lasting change.

I've never considered myself a seller of ideas, but a teacher of concepts. These concepts are contained in the pages of this book and provide the map to take steps on your journey from where you are now to where you want to be. My role in this process is to be your guide—a guide with a good map to show you the way.

The purpose of this book is to **CHANGE YOUR LIFE.** If you follow these concepts and principles, you will have success and create lasting change within you. These principles can help you in all areas of your life, so it's really just a matter of how much change and how soon it will come with your commitment to learning.

I learned a long time ago that there is a price to pay for everything—and you must be willing to pay that price. In this case, it's following these principles and committing yourself to applying them in your daily life. If you find yourself initially not wanting to pay a price for changing then remember this: There is always a price to pay for changing and a price to pay for staying the same. You're already paying that price, the real trick is, to have fun paying the price—you will learn how to focus on what you want and add as much positive emotion to it as you can. If you're unwilling to pay the price, let it be okay that you are staying the same.

REMEMBER THAT IF IT IS IMPORTANT TO YOU, YOU WILL FIND A WAY.

IF NOT, YOU'LL FIND AN EXCUSE.

Sometimes, we are not ready to pay the price or we are too emotionally bankrupt to afford it. That's okay too. You have taken the first step of considering change. You can take another step and move ahead when you are ready. The day will come when you are ready because the pain of staying the same will be worse than the pain of changing.

What you are learning is not a set of rules you need to follow in order to achieve a specific goal of losing weight. In fact, what you are learning is how to transform yourself from the inside out. Each chapter will give you the tools, strategies and action points for you to make these changes to the way you think, and feel and this will change your behavior.

Be willing to be open to the ideas that are presented here. You may even wonder what any of this has to do with you losing weight. The point is that the first shift in your perception must be that your goal to lose weight is secondary to you changing your relationship with yourself and with food. If you solely focus on behavior and rule-based eating that diets teach, you will only have success as long as you are following these rules.

In Chapter 1 you will learn why dieting doesn't work and this is the start to you breaking the eat, guilt, repent, repeat cycle. If you've ever felt like you are a failure and that you will never lose weight then here's where the rubber meets the road. You did not fail, the diet failed you. Hitting the preverbal diet bottom is a good thing, because only from here can you shed that tiny amount of hope you cling to that THIS will be the diet that does it. You know what I mean and we've all been there. You're all hyped up and ready to begin the new weight loss plan that promises so much. This will be the diet that changes everything! You will have that rocking body. You will get that promotion! You will buy a new wardrobe! You will have that fulfilling and sextacular relationship you've always desired! You'll be at the gym everyday showing off your new svelte form. You will walk out into the world with your head held high and everyone will be looking at you wondering what your secret is. You will be the envy of all. You'll be sharing your story to the world! Everyone will want to know how you did it. That old boyfriend of yours who dumped you? He's eating his heart out and you couldn't be happier. You'll feel that elated sense of confidence that you've got it now. You will have the life you've always dreamed of. Everything will be great.

Your motivation is high, your determination is strong and you set out with the greatest of intentions. With fierce enthusiasm you start out on your new plan and are steadfast and true to the letter. It feels good to have structure. You know what you need to eat and not to eat. You know you can have a certain amount of calories each day. You can drink two shakes and you can eat a sensible meal each day. It's so easy as all the meals will be delivered to your door and their chefs have prepared everything for you! You can lose the weight and keep it off! Watching your weight has never been easier with pro points because it works! You've cut out carbs, wheat, dairy and you are eating clean. You know everything there is to know about food combining and weigh out everything. It's time to stop dieting and start living, one point at a time. You can fight the trend of obesity starting with yourself and be a product of the product. All you have to do is follow this plan by living it, eating it, sleeping it and repeating it. Your diet is your life.

After the first week, you begin to notice a difference as you weigh yourself on the scale the same time every day and you feel encouraged. After the second week, you've lost even more weight and people have begun to notice. You feel strong! You feel confident! There was that one day, when you had that cake, but you won't tell anyone. To others, you are a monument of willpower and discipline. People test you by offering you extra portions and treats. You easily dismiss this attempt to derail you. You are a fortress!

By the third week, you've begun to feel a bit weak. Your body feels tired and you put this down to the detox your body is going through. Sure, there are the occasional headaches and fatigue, but you know this will pass. You find yourself thinking of food most of the time. Your structured eating approach works, but you cannot stop thinking about cake! The more you try not to think about cake, the more you think about cake and you're beginning to lose your mind. You go to the gym to purge your food demons.

You have a bad day. Work was terrible. You argued with your husband. You feel awful. You cannot face another shake. All you want is a chocolate bar dipped in mayonnaise, wrapped in bacon, deep fried with syrup on it. You're tired. You're sick. You're sick and tired and tired of being sick. You breakdown and have an almighty binge. You wallow in all the foods you have denied yourself and you go back for seconds and thirds. As long as you continue to eat, you won't feel that way. So you keep eating. Eating and eating until you cannot eat anymore. Here, at the bottom of every empty bag or container, you meet yourself. You are a failure. You've done it again. Why did you do that? You are weak. You are no good. You will never be happy. You don't deserve happiness anyways. You cry yourself to sleep with a bulging gut, heavy heart and a guilt-ridden mind.

The next day, you throw away your resolve as it's the weekend. You might as well have the next few days to get this out of your system. Once it's out of your system, you'll resolve and repent and get back on track. You've not attended the gym and the following week, after eating like it was going out of fashion, your body feels sluggish and the last thing you want to do is waddle it up and down on the elliptical trainer.

Sound familiar?

Step by step you will be peeling back the layers of years of conditioning to expose the truth that lies within. So far, you've been running on automatic, making choices to the best of your current knowledge. This book will give you strategies and tools to assist you in breaking through all the junk in your mental trunk to expose who you really are, what you really need and what you can do to achieve it.

In Chapter 2 you will be learning why making peace with your body is crucial to your transformation. So many people are at war with themselves. They make change a problem. Change can lead to uncertainty and in my experience, people would rather be certain and unhappy than to try something new and feel uncertain.

There's a lot of buzz around the 'health at every size' movement and it really is wonderful that people are beginning to understand body diversity. Acceptance of your body doesn't mean you've resigned yourself to being a larger size. What it means is that you put your health as a priority and you are taking responsibility for your transformation. It enables you to give up on excuses and embrace everything about yourself.

Transformation comes from taking consistent action steps that lead you to the change. The recommendations in this book are not 'drastic, fat melting, weight loss is everything and who gives a poop about your health as long as you are skinny' steps. It's about taking deliberate action toward where you really want to go. If you do not want love, happiness, acceptance and joy for yourself and your body, then you can pass this book along to a friend right now.

In Chapter 3 you will make peace with food. How long has food been the enemy? How long have you been avoiding certain foods? If you have been restricting and depriving yourself as a means to achieve your desired weight then it's time to reset this relationship to NEUTRAL.

You will be challenged to consider how you've developed your relationship with food through your family growing up, through others and of course, through chronic dieting.

I have yet to meet a client who doesn't have a distorted and disordered eating approach based on years and years of dieting. They know the calorie count of every chocolate bar. They can tell you just as quick how many hours they would need in the gym to work it off. They pride themselves as being a walking encyclopedia of diet information and could probably write their own book!

They have lost hundreds of pounds of weight over the years and have put it back on again. They never consider where they may have learned to eat the way they do or how their past could have affected their relationship with food. Like 'clean plate syndrome'. So many of my clients feel they must eat everything on their plate or else they feel they've wasted it. They've learned to cook for an army of people when there is only a few to feed. They starve themselves all day in a bid to be good so by the time they get home they could eat the tail end of a rabid donkey and still want to go back for seconds or thirds!

Transformation starts as an inside job. It is an internal game which begins with your thoughts. In Chapter 4 you will be exploring the most powerful resource you have: Your imagination. Everything you do or don't do depends on thinking. You can imagine yourself in all kinds of scenarios and if you are in the habit of thinking about everything you do not want, you will act and react in a way to self fulfill this. Everything you think is an affirmation. When you affirm it over and over again, it becomes wired into your neurology as a belief.

The majority of people walk around in a perpetual sleepwalk. They coast through life on autopilot being reactive to everything. Thoughts come and go again. They never really consider choosing their thoughts or intentionally thinking about things based on what they want. They bumble around from experience to experience letting life shape them, instead of living creatively and intentionally. In order to break out of this trance like state, you need to wake up and understand the power of your thoughts and the power of your mind to create positive change.

All the behaviors and habits you have are because you've learned how to do them. All behaviors have a purpose and you can unlearn them. This starts with understanding the mind, the language of the mind and how you can affect positive change through your thinking.

In Chapter 5 you will learn how some beliefs are like hardwired thoughts you will need to uninstall for transformation. Before I became a therapist, I was a marketing professional. This was not by design but by default. I was sleepwalking as well. I ended up in this profession as life carried me from job to job, place to place, experience to experience and relationship to relationship. It was indeed my struggle and my unhappiness that helped me to wake up. I was desperately unhappy. I was depressed and unfulfilled. I blamed my childhood for most of my problems. I had terrible coping mechanisms. I drank too much to escape myself only to end up feeling worse later on.

Life was hard. Every day I woke up feeling dread. I managed to shake it off and just get on with it as I felt I just had to suck it up. I did this for many, many years. Until one day, desperate for change, I went seeking something different. I took a leap of faith and began to open myself up to new ideas. Life seemed to greet me with new possibilities. In the Wizard of Oz, Dorothy was urged to follow the yellow brick road. Dorothy, like me, was unhappy with her current situation and despite the familiarity of life in Kansas, she wondered what was over the rainbow.

The discontent I felt put me into action. I began to search for my life and awaken to the possibilities. Books seemed to leap off the shelf and from one book in particular, I began my transformation. The book was called Dante's Path: A Practical Approach to Achieving Inner Wisdom by Bonney Gulino and Richard Schaub.

I remember how I found the book, or how the book found me. I was surfing the web and searched 'gaining confidence for self esteem'. A link appeared for EBay and in the search results was this book. It wasn't specifically about self esteem or confidence, but it resonated with me. So I purchased it.

In my search for more confidence and self esteem I found myself being guided to something even more profound: My own transformation. As I sat with this book recently, I noticed many corners of it turned down for reference. I hadn't looked at this book for about 10 years. I opened the book to a referenced page where there is a title called The Three Choices; "Once you grasp the reality of your actual vulnerable situation, you have three choices. The first is to try to escape from reality, the second is to try to gain power over it, and the third is to study it in more depth by going on a spiritual journey. Every one of us, as human beings, has made each one of these choices at some time in our life. There's nothing wrong with that, either, unless we begin to rely exclusively on either escape or power as the answer to our fears, because neither escape nor power is capable of producing an enduring antidote to our basic fear."

The book itself draws on Dante's epic poem The Divine Comedy as a rich metaphor for the challenge of escaping from fear-based instincts (Dante's Hell); into a place of personal transformation (Purgatory), then into the confidence of finding life's higher purpose (his Pilgrim's Paradise). The reader is taken through the metaphor with insights as a map to move out of our personal hell through improving the quality of our consciousness.

This was the first time I had come across the ideas presented in this book, but it didn't shock me. I had been in the habit for many years of dismissing such spiritual concepts as 'new age'. That didn't happen with this. The book spoke directly to me and I identified with the circles of hell described as indifference, addiction and greed. The goal of indifference is to feel nothing; the goal of addiction is to feel soothed; and the goal of greed is to feel invulnerable and secure.

The goal of this book is to improve the quality of your consciousness by becoming aware and directing your consciousness energetically. You become the witness who has the ability to name but not shame what they are aware of. It is a non-judgemental curiosity that is cultivated. Discovering what beliefs you hold about yourself, your life and your place in this world is the place I started. From there, the layers peeled back to expose more and more truths that were hidden under the conditioned certainty and discomfort of the blankets I slept beneath.

Often, a person has to reach some sort of impasse in their life to spur them to begin their own spiritual journey much like Dorothy confronted her own demons "lions and tigers and bears, oh my!"

For me, it was leaving behind what I believed to be true about myself based on experiences of my childhood and challenging myself to know who I would be without that. What I have learned is that I am only limited by what I believe is possible.

In Chapter 6 we explore how to apply intention creatively by taking action. I really wanted to dispel the magical element that is applied to manifesting your dreams. The word manifesting conjures up the idea there's some sort of magic to being able to be the creative force in your life. Again, this brings up the power of the guru / coach / therapist / whatever they call themselves, to change you. They have found the miraculous and magical manifestation secrets and for $999 you can learn how to use them to manifest your dream relationship, your dream car, your perfect body, your million dollar lifestyle complete with your happiness and fulfillment.

I cannot over emphasize how shallow it is to think that by using your imagination you will attract to you all the riches you feel you lack right now. Fundamentally, you don't attract what you want, you attract what you are. If you are lacking, you attract lack. You must FEEL your way to your goals. Whatever you want in life is on the other side of your fears. You must first dismantle the inner workings of your beliefs, values and conditioned mindset in order to create the life you feel you deserve.

With all of this transformation happening, Chapter 7 shows you how to deal with the chaos that creating these types of changes will bring up inside of you. What do I mean by chaos? When you are making changes at a deep level of understanding it will feel as though your whole world if falling apart. That is because it is. The internal world that you've created in your beliefs, values, perceptions, attitudes, habits and strategies that have created your experience of life.

If you anticipate there will be some discomfort in making change, but that it's part of the process, it's easier to face. It will also help you to recognize the signs of change and to lean into it. It is only temporary but all complex systems go through this process.

I wanted to also address the matter of quitting. I know a lot of my clients give up on the process. It's important to understand that this is your life and there really is no quitting until it's the end of your life. We have a tendency to think we have unlimited time to try and quit and try again, but frankly, we don't know when the end of our time will be. I want you to appreciate that you cannot quit until you quit living your life.

If you were to live every moment of your life to the fullest because you believed you were worth it and appreciated all that you have right now, you'd be living in the now. In Chapter 8 I address how we waste our precious moments living in the past or in the future, rarely living in the now.

As the quality of your consciousness changes, you will appreciate your present moments even more. You'll be taking action which empowers you to make choices to support the healthiest you. You'll feel happier, more energized and more alive than you ever have. With your increasing ability to witness and name your experience, you can get out in front of problems before they even happen. With practice a peaceful strength will be with you throughout your daily life.

This would not be possible for you if you didn't let go of your negative past. In Chapter 9 we address how the past influences our present moment. When you begin to appreciate how you've lived according to what you believed was true, how your story affects everything about your perception of life, and with your newly cultivated quality consciousness, you can transform your story.

For my clients and for me, this means you no longer identify with the stories you've told yourself and others thousands of times throughout your life. Who would you be if you didn't believe that? What would happen if you woke up one day and you didn't remember anything about who you were before that moment?

Some may be terrified, defensive or confused by such a prospect. The point is that you are the person who applies the meaning and even if you've inherited that meaning, you are the only one who can change it to mean something that supports you making positive changes in your life.

We wear our pain like a badge of honor. We feel we are what we were. The only thing you need to be certain of is that you can be whatever you want yourself to be and this does not need to be defined by who you were.

This will mean you need to forgive others and even yourself. In Chapter 10 we look at what forgiveness is and how you can use it to shed the weight of your negative past. Everyone has been hurt at some point in their life. Everyone has baggage. The point is that if your baggage is weighing you down and you are carrying a lot of resentment and bitterness, your progress will be stifled by this. It is only when we are truly free from the burden of the perceived injustices that we are free to live life fully to our potentials. Sometimes we need the hurt, pain and betrayal in order for us to wake up to ourselves.

If someone goes through their life never having met challenges, they never really grow. You may know someone who is very pampered or spoiled. If someone has never had to deal with consequences, is always bailed out or never pushed out of their comfort zones, they stay at the same emotional level. People with the most emotional intelligence and resilience are those who have experienced and overcome struggles. By changing the way you look at the 'bad' things that have happened to you and by understanding that everyone is doing the best they can at their current level of consciousness you can be compassionate towards everyone. This really takes the sting out of experiences and allows you to move forward stronger and healthier without the poison in your mind and body hindering your progress.

You may need to forgive in order to move forward. This may mean forgiving yourself. You may have spent a lot of time in your life beating yourself up because you've not been able to make the changes you think will make you happy. In order to move forward so you can create true happiness and joy in your life you need to be kind to yourself. Learning to practice self compassion gives you permission to be a spiritual being having a human experience on your journey of self growth.

If you had an attitude where you were grateful for everything in your life how do you think this would transform your experience? If you no longer felt like your life lacked some quality or experience how would you feel about yourself and your life? If you weren't envious of others and felt inadequate in some way how would that be for you? In Chapter 11 you will learn the power of being grateful for everything in your life. There is nothing wrong with wanting more in your life, however, if by wanting more you feel there is something lacking and that you cannot be happy until you fill the void you will always be searching for something. When you get that something it will not be enough. If you do feel fulfilled it will only be momentarily as there will always be something you seek outside of yourself to fill your void. The only way to fill the void is to be grateful with everything you already have. The most important thing in life is to recognize that it is not things we need to feel complete.

During this process of transformation you will experience lots of feelings. Chapter 12 shares with you tools and strategies for dealing with uncomfortable emotions without using food. You can begin to appreciate that your feelings are the way your body communicates with you. When you learn to listen and feel your way through your life, you will not be guided wrongly. Your body has a wisdom that will assist you, if you get out of its way and let your body do what it knows how to do.

So far, the book has explored the inner workings of your transformation. It is the thoughts and feelings of how your inner world creates your experience of life. You've looked at your emotional and psychological needs and probably have a better understanding about them. The priority is always on healing the self and making whole what was incomplete. Without that, any attempt to change your physical appearance by only changing your behaviors will be short-term. Chapter 13 introduces the principles and philosophies of Intuitive Eating.

With your understanding of these principles, you can bring together all that you've learned and adopt into your life a new approach to eating mindfully according to your body's needs. You will also explore some common hurdles in adopting a new approach like diet bonding and creating balance.

Chapter 14 will address the excuses associated with moving your body to help you change your perspective on activity. It's essential you understand that what you are aiming at achieving is a balanced, healthy lifestyle. Moving your body feels good and doing so is not a remedy or punishment for being fat.

The final chapters in the book will help you to embrace the process of transformation. To understand that this is your life, not a quick fix to a long term solution so that you can commit to this transformation for the right reasons.

As you set out on this journey from where you are to where you want to be, consider the lessons in this book as a guide pointing you in the right direction towards beginning this transformation. Trust in the process of life to move you forward to where your soul wants you to be. Allow yourself to be empowered and don't be afraid of your emerging strength as you awaken from your sleepwalk state, release old wounds and heal your internal world to expose the highest expression of yourself. What you will gain is the courage and confidence to make any changes you want in your life.

I have experienced this transformation in myself and seen it in my clients. When you can let go of excuses and fear-based agendas that keep you stuck you transcend your current reality and embrace what your wisest self has planned for your life.

It's always a choice and you've already made the choice to read this book. Your transformation is waiting.

Chapter 1—Hitting Diet Bottom

"I keep trying to lose weight, but it keeps finding me!"
~ Author Unknown

Did you know that diets have a 95% failure rate? The diet industry is a multi-billion dollar industry. You need to ask yourself that IF diets did work, then surely this industry wouldn't be as successful as it is. Research suggests that during a lifetime people spend 30 years on diets, the average length of each attempt is just over five weeks long before throwing in the towel due to the regimented fatigue of restriction leaving the person moody and depressed.

Diets are about restriction, limitation and deprivation. They only work when you are doing them and it's hard work. It's a real effort to count calories and make healthier choices. This restriction creates a mentality of "I can't" / "I shouldn't".

When we are in this mentality, we find it difficult to avoid thinking of all the food we can't have. Don't think of chocolate biscuits. Don't think of them! What happens, the more you try not to think about them, the more you do. This is because the mind thinks in images and representations of things, making it impossible to not think about exactly what you do not want to think about.

The rigidness of diets means you can only do them for a short period of time before you get bored, rebel or just give up because of the exhaustive effort of applying the rules. This internal struggle is like fighting against yourself and your thoughts to avoid when you inevitably cave in. Then you feel guilty or a failure because of all those things you could not / should not have had.

Frankly, dieting is a form of starvation which triggers a biological / chemical response in us to crave more food. Traci Mann, associate professor of the UCLA has reported in the American

Psychological Association's journal *American Psychologist* that "You can initially lose 5 to 10 percent of your weight on any number of diets, but then the weight comes back. Diets do not lead to sustained weight loss or health benefits for the majority of people."

In analyzing the data of hundreds of weight loss studies which took place over a 2 to 5 year period, researchers concluded that most people would have been better off not going on the diet at all as their weight was pretty much the same, except for the wear and tear their body suffered from losing weight and gaining it all back again.

Dieting damages the body, the mind and the spirit. Have you ever felt like a complete failure after yet another diet disaster? Your self esteem and trust in yourself erodes with each feeble attempt to outsmart your biology. The truth is you didn't fail, the diet failed because your biology will win every time.

The assertion of your autonomy will prevail, as it is greater than your desire to lose weight, since a diet creates an internal violation to your body's primal biological directives: **TO STAY ALIVE**.

The human body is an amazing and complex system, and nearly perfect in the way it is set up to run. However, people learn to ignore their bodies and deny the natural flow of maintaining a default, healthy natural weight for themselves.

Hormones play an important role in weight loss / management and Lubert Stryer, Professor of Biochemistry at Stanford University cited that our metabolism of energy utilization essentially is the responsibility of two pancreatic proteins: glucagon for weight loss and insulin for weight gain. These hormones being in balance is essential for healthy metabolism.

These hormones (and others) regulate your body's weight management. Basically, they are behind your hunger and satiety cues and are there to protect you (keep you alive). When dieting, your biological systems will attempt to correct this mistake by stimulating hunger and appetite so you feel hungry all the time.

The dieter uses their 'willpower' as a way to follow rules to attempt to counter physiological signals by ignoring or suppressing hunger cues to the point of atrophy. Your body will decrease metabolic processing of energy as a way to reserve / ration out the energy, otherwise known as 'fasting mode'. In this mode, research shows that prolonged fasting leads the body into starvation mode, where the insulin levels are spiked so whatever is eaten is stored as fat. Your fat cells are the reserves for your body to avoid starvation. Being in starvation mode makes you more susceptible to craving foods which are higher in calories and denser in fat. It's a lose-lose situation.

Every dieter knows that food becomes so seductive to them, that when they do eat, it is an intense experience that is prone to over indulging or a sense of entitlement as they become desperate and insatiable in their eating behavior.

At 48 Sally lost 55 pounds of weight following a strict calorie restrictive plan of two shakes per day, one snack bar and a "sensible dinner" of no more than 1200 calories per day over a four month period. She experienced a lot of ups and downs during this time and cheated on her diet now and again, but picked herself back up and remounted her diet saddle after each subsequent relapse. She came to see me because she still hadn't reached her goal of losing 75 pounds. She was tired of drinking her meals and wanted to find a better way. This was one of her many attempts to lose this weight over the course of 20 years and she was desperate to make it work this time.

She was a busy executive and juggled work with her home life. Her children were out of the house and it was just her and her husband living at home. After a busy day at the office, where she found it easy to stick to her regimented diet, home life proved a terrifying and difficult struggle for her.

Her husband was an excellent cook and enjoyed expressing his love through food. The whole process for him was a way to show he cared. Unfortunately, Sally had very few foods she was allowed to eat. Her self-imposed eating rules meant once she was home, she was bombarded with the sights, smells and temptations of a passionate foodie. She loathed coming home and pleaded with her husband to ensure he made lighter choices such as lean protein with steamed vegetables and perhaps some brown rice or quiona. Basically, she was a food saint being lured into food hell by her devil of a husband and she blamed him for her diet failures. She told me "If only he didn't cook those foods then I wouldn't be tempted and I could lose the weight."

On the days where she stayed strong, she would eat with full entitlement every last crumb and practically lick the plate clean as if it was the last supper she would ever eat. If she was feeling weak after an especially stressful day, she would throw her diet into the wind and eat everything in sight plus seconds or thirds. What she failed to understand was that it wasn't her husband, his cooking, her stress, or even the food that was the cause of her succumbing to the whims of her ferocious appetite, it was her biology. Physiologically her body is programmed to meet its basic biological needs and you cannot out will or out think your biology.

Like Sally, dieters find themselves in this cycle of failure where deprivation leads to cravings, which leads to compulsive and intrusive thoughts about food, creating more desire for eating. When they do give in to their biology, they feel out of control, guilt, shame and it erodes their trust in themselves around food as they begin to believe "there's something wrong with me."

There is nothing wrong with you! This is a normal response to starvation!

In a breakthrough study called "The Biology of Human Starvation" by Ancel Keys, thirty-six college aged men who were healthy were put on diets of half their normal daily calorie intake (approximately 1200 calories per day) for six months, to astonishing findings:

Participants demonstrated a preoccupation with food. They talked about it and their interests included gathering and sharing recipes (these are post-war men living in the 1940s!). Their cravings were heightened and they had less fussy eating—the foods they used to dislike they began to consider! They became stingy and possessive about their food and didn't want to share.

During the study, some of the men escaped and had a food eating frenzy at a local food store where they binged, vomited and felt intense feelings of guilt. This sounds very much like the beginning signs of an eating disorder!

Personality changes included apathy and bouts of depression described as feeling 'useless'. They lost interest in sex and other interests and two subjects are cited as 'bordering on psychoses including violent outbursts and hysteria'.

Physical changes show they had slower pulse rate, their basic metabolic rate reduced 40% and participants felt slower and behaved older. Generally, they were unhappy in mood and lost their sense of humor or it became sarcastic in tone. They were reluctant to participate in social and group activities.

They became withdrawn, isolated and unable to control their emotional states.

During the re-feeding stage where the men were given limited access to food, and this was followed by unlimited access to food, the effects noted that their appetites were insatiable even on the highest caloric levels allowed. They continued to eat even when stuffed; they ate on average 5,212 kcal when given free access to food and gained fat tissue rapidly.

Chronic dieting causes the body to change shape so more fat is stored around the middle / stomach area. Metabolism slows with each diet, making it harder and harder to shift with each subsequent diet attempt. More and more fat is stored as a form of self preservation, making it harder and harder to lose. In order to get your body into balance so you burn stored fat, you need to kick in the fat burning hormone. If your body is a vehicle, then insulin is a gas pipe from the fuel tank to the engine, which is glucagon.

The problem is, people are so engrained into the diet mentality they don't know when they are hungry because they've become so adept at ignoring the signals their body is communicating or they eat when they think they should: "It's lunchtime, better get something to eat." But are you hungry? Do you know what genuine, biological hunger feels like?

If you imagine that your body is a machine, you need to tune it up, start your engine, burn fuel and for weight loss this is the reserved fuel you've stored in your fat cells. By listening to your body, eating when you are hungry and *only when you are hungry,* you are working with your body, listening and responding to the natural signals of hunger and satisfaction.

Optimal fat loss is achieved when you are in this flow. Naturally the human body will begin to crave food after 3 to 4 hours between the last food intake, and this is where the magic happens. Hunger is **GOLD**! And you can feed your hunger with food and slim! I realize that diets are about limitation, deprivation and restriction, but the fact is they hinder your progress of slimming, creating unhealthy associations with food and patterns of eating which work out of alignment with your body's natural flow.

By paying attention to your body's natural sensory cues of hunger you are able to retrain yourself and get your body and mind back in balance. For example, at night, when sleeping we go into fasting mode. This slows down our digestive system to allow that energy to be expended in other more essential tasks whilst the body rests. This is why we do not get hungry during our slumber. When you awake you may not be feeling the sensation of hunger because you are still in fasting mode. Think about the word breakfast = BREAK FAST. You need to break the fast to stoke the fire of your metabolism with fuel. Food is fuel. From that point on, if you listen to your vehicle (your body) you will hear it telling you when it's time for more fuel.

That's right, eating is encouraged and allowed! In fact, the only fully scientifically supported appetite suppressant available is none other than **FOOD**! Makes sense doesn't it? In order to liberate yourself from the cycle of chronic dieting, overeating and yo-yo weight fluctuations, you need to tune into your body and eat intuitively.

The key principle to eating intuitively is about getting back in rapport with your body. To listen, understand and respond to the many ways your body lets you know it's time to eat and when you've had enough. As a result, intuitive eaters are able to retain their healthy, default, natural weight effortlessly. This means you need to work from the inside-out and this starts with changing what you've learned so far. You came into this world eating intuitively according to the natural rhythm of your hunger and satiety cycles and along the way you've learned differently. You became out of touch with your body, your feelings and yourself. You've learned to ignore what you want and desire, and put in its place things you think you should want and eat or shouldn't want and don't eat.

This book is here to teach you how to become the expert of yourself. You already know yourself better than anyone else. So you need to learn to trust in yourself to distinguish between emotional and physical hunger and respond accordingly. You can return to eating without struggle, guilt, deprivation or obsession with food. If you were to eat based on internal signals of biological hunger instead of external signals of schedule, time, stress or other triggers you would be able to return to your body's natural weight and maintain it. This means you will need to unlearn and relearn how to do this. This is more than just a book about eating intuitively and mindfully, you will also examine the emotional, psychological, physical, biological and spiritual components to transform your relationship with yourself, food and your life. This book shows you how to change from the inside out.

Emotional overeating is the number one cause of obesity, yet diet plans fail to address this fact. This is because diets only address the symptoms of overeating (weight gain, for example), not the underlying reasons. With a diet, you let the diet tell you when and what to eat and you rely on willpower to get you through it. In almost all cases, willpower cannot last for long as deprivation kicks in, which leads to overeating and weight gain. You eat too much if you had a bad day, you are stressed, you are sad, you are lonely or bored. Perhaps you're happy, you've had a great day, and you are going to celebrate so you treat yourself by over indulging. Either way, you are using food as a salve or reward and this can create a cycle of behavior that may seem impossible to break free from.

"You are my only hope; I am desperate." Karen was almost in tears when she confessed she was a chronic dieter. From the time of 8 years old she was on and off diets from the cabbage diet, to diet pills, slimming clubs and liquid shakes. Now at age 46 she was at her largest size and weight, her self esteem had rotted away with her countless dieting disasters.

Karen was convinced that if this approach didn't work for her, nothing would and she'd have to settle with feeling terrible about herself, become even more isolated socially and get bigger and fatter. When discussing her expectations it became clear that what she wanted was a quick-fix that I was unable to deliver.

"Just make me stop eating the wrong foods and make me feel full all the time and then I'll be happy," she begged with a red-eyed innocence.

This is a very common theme with my clients seeking weight loss. They think that if they have A, then that will bring them B, which will equal C, happiness. Actually the equation would look like this:

A: Eat the "right" foods + B: Feel full and satisfied = C : I'm slim—which means I am happy!

At this point I always ask my clients if they have ever been slim in their life. Most can remember a time where they were a size smaller then they are now. The paradox about it is, when I ask if they were happy with their bodies at that time, most say they were not. They thought they were fat even then and wanted to slim. This most likely happened as they or an associate compared themselves to someone else and in this comparison they began to look at their bodies differently—as if they were wrong and needed fixing, and this is when they began their lifetime struggle with dieting.

The truth is you are not your size. You, like me, probably know thin, miserable people. Maybe in your thinner days, you were one of them. They are slim, but unhappy and unfulfilled. They are critical of themselves and always feel like they need to change.

"Happiness is not a goal; it is a by-product." Eleanor Roosevelt

In a breakthrough study where 10 years of data was analyzed, the *National Growth and Health Study* looking at the attitudes of two groups of over 2,000 black and white women towards their bodies found that even after they lost weight, their self-esteem remained low. Furthermore, despite their lower body mass index, both groups continued to have negative body perceptions. The conclusion was that the body image of both groups of women in the study did not rebound as the stigma about their size still lingered.

Purdue sociology researcher, Sarah Mustillo concluded that, "Body image is so tied up with our overall sense of self. So when we look in the mirror and feel deficient, or look at another woman and feel 'less than', it isn't just about body. It's about a deeper sense of unworthiness, and that just gets expressed in the body.

"On a fundamental level, compassion for ourselves and others, and connectedness with others, might improve body image. It is helpful to remember that underneath all our physical differences, we're all emotional beings with needs and insecurities."

When chasing the holy grail of the 'perfect size', the 'perfect body' in the wish to have the 'perfect life', we are chasing an illusion which can never be realized. Just as much as happiness is not some place you arrive at one day after trying hard to find it. This is where the veils begin to lift and the client begins to see that the way they have been searching for their solution is the biggest component to creating their problem.

At this point, reassurance is needed for them to understand that the priority for making this change is an inside job. What this means is that the key to making positive changes lies in the relationship we have with ourselves and our food.

So what is your relationship with yourself? Ask yourself: Do I love and accept myself just as I am?

If the answer is no, then you have a poor relationship with yourself. A poor relationship with yourself is most often about negative body perceptions or self image. This negative self image is the way you see yourself, whether through your judgemental eye or as perceived by the eyes of the world demonstrated as lack of self confidence or self consciousness. Perhaps you have negative self talk and focus on everything you dislike about the way your body looks and call yourself names. Do you look in the mirror and dislike what you see?

This poor relationship is a hindrance in moving forward in a positive way in your life. Why would you do something that is going to create a positive change if you don't like who you are or what you look like?

It is a catch 22 cycle. You are unhappy with yourself, you want to change. You have a poor relationship with food that has developed over many years of conditioning. You turn to food as a salve for feeling awful in yourself and then beat yourself up afterwards with feelings of guilt or shame. Then you resolve and repent, with a solemn promise to never do it again and tell yourself that 'this time will be different' and start the cycle all over again.

Love and acceptance in your relationship with yourself needs to take precedence before any other relationships can be healed. When you are able to love what you see, feel great knowing you are making improvements and changes and love yourself for doing so, then you are pressing down on the accelerator to get you from where you are to where you want to go.

A healthy relationship comes from healing our pasts. We were all born into this world perfect and adoring ourselves. We had confidence and we believed ourselves worthy of good things. It's only in experiences of our life and interactions with others we are told things that are not true, and we believe them.

To break the cycle it takes courage to take responsibility for yourself. Otherwise, you will be a victim of yourself, your life and the experiences of your past. The first step is in understanding you need to own this change by taking responsibility for all the choices you made before, all the choices you make now and the choices you make in the future.

It is a process or a journey and like any journey, there's a beginning and an ending. Along the way there will be detours, challenges, obstacles and other lessons you can use as feedback for your growth. That is all there is: life and you're living it, right now. The priority is changing your relationship with yourself, your body and with food. This is where you start. As you read through each chapter of this book, you will take further steps in making all these changes towards transformation.

Action Steps:

1. Make a decision right now to stop dieting.

2. Make healing your relationship with yourself and with food a priority.

3. Commit yourself to the process of transformation.

Chapter 2—The Gift of Acceptance

"The curious paradoxis that when I accept myself just as I am, then I can change."
~ Carl Rogers, American psychologist

Many of my clients have made a distinction between the way they look and who they are. Basically, they hate the way they look and although they 'like' themselves as people, they hate and loathe their bodies. Body-bashing becomes the acceptable norm.

They've fallen out of love with themselves. This is not the arrogant 'I love myself' type of adoration. This is the natural self love that every human born into the world has. It is the wide-eyed and wondrous curiosity about themselves and their world. Babies do not make a distinction between themselves and everything else. We learn that there is 'us' and 'them' or one thing and another thing in our developmental perception as we get older. We also learn how to relate to ourselves through the interactions we have with others.

Body assessment and comparison has become the obsessive pastime of the chronic dieter. Rarely, are my clients concerned with how things 'feel' to them but are quick to focus on how things 'look' to them. Their confidence and mood is directly influenced by what the scales are reading. If the scales show they've lost weight, they are happy. If not, well, they are frustrated and agitated with themselves. This could be another failed attempt, another notch up on the chronic dieter's belt.

Christina was obsessed with comparing herself to others. Weight loss had become a sport. She revelled in her weekly weigh-ins at her local slimming support group. It really lit a fire in her belly to beat the other women each week. Of course, outwardly, she was sympathetic, reassuring and even commiserated their lack of loss, but inwardly, she got satisfaction from their failure. This went on for a couple of months until she returned from holiday where she had 'fallen off the diet wagon'. She felt too ashamed of her weight gain so she didn't attend her slimming support group until she had returned to the weight she was before (plus a bit) so she could brag about her success to the group.

We live in an image-obsessed culture that respects cultural diversity but still has trouble with body diversity. We all come in different shapes, sizes and structures but get a distorted perspective that we should all be one-size-fits-all. This narrow perspective may be aggravated by an idealization of the physical form, which is promoted by celebrity and media hype. My clients all understand that what they see in magazines and in the media is an enhanced and unrealistic interpretation of the diversity of the human form, but dismiss it just as easily. The truth is there are no perfect bodies, perfect bodies are not real and real bodies are not perfect!

Overweight people are seen to be less attractive, less capable and weaker in character than their slimmer counterparts. Slim is seen as successful, capable and attractive. It is important to recognize there are many factors in determining body size which includes diet, eating patterns, genetics, activity level, health factors and nutrition. This prejudice does not start or end with slim people observing overweight people; it comes from everywhere including the chronic dieter as they hold judgement against themselves. The unfortunate truth is that you cannot assume that just because someone is slimmer that they got there in a healthy way. Nor can you assume that because someone is heavier that they got there in an unhealthy way.

There is a biological, genetic, natural weight that is right for us. When you clear out misconceptions, assumptions, judgements and negativity held in the mind towards yourself or others you begin to return to this default weight that is right for you—naturally. The reality is, it may not be the fashionably slim size 4 you may have been hoping for, but it will be what is right for you. Just as much as you wouldn't expect a size 7 foot to fit into a size 5 shoe, you can begin to accept yourself and feel better about yourself, the whole you.

A positive relationship with ourselves is the key essential step and can be one of the most difficult for my clients to heal. Ask yourself: "Do I love and accept myself just as I am?"

Love and acceptance for yourself is key to making any positive change. If you find yourself not being able to honestly say you do, then it's time to work on that. Let's define what is meant by acceptance:

Acceptance in this definition does not mean approval. It means acknowledgement. It does not mean you are submitting or resigning either. It is about responsibility—and responsibility does not mean placing blame or fault. It is about being empowered to make better choices for yourself from this moment into all your other future moments.

Most people will think acceptance means approval. Does this sound familiar? "If I approve of myself, it means I do not have a problem. That means I will continue to get fatter and bigger. I want to change and be slimmer. So, in order to be motivated, I will not approve of myself."

ACCEPTANCE IS ABOUT CHANGE. It says: "I'm ready to change. I am willing and I take 100% responsibility for where I am now." It's an acknowledgement of where you are now. It marks you clearly on your map of change. It enables you to claim that "this is where I am right now, my current weight, size, shape, attitude, beliefs, feelings, thoughts, eating behaviors, excuses and all the accumulation of all the choices I ever made which led me to this perfect moment."

If you are still struggling to accept yourself just as you are under this definition remember, without acceptance just as you are, you will find it difficult to plan your journey to where you want to be. It's as if you go to set off on a journey from New York and you want to go to Los Angeles by car but you do not accept the fact you are in New York to begin with. How are you going to begin to plan your journey if you do not accept where you are right now?

Acceptance does not mean approval. It means acknowledgement and responsibility. It's right you want to make improvements and changes. That is a positive choice. You do not have to withhold acceptance for yourself to make a positive choice and to change. In fact, by accepting yourself just as you are you can be clear where you are and set out to where you want to go with even more conviction and clarity.

So, with that definition, can you now accept yourself just as you are? Consider how you can and what that means.

You do not have to make the size you are a problem. In fact, making it a problem is part of the problem. Think about it like this: by being down on yourself, withholding love and acceptance for yourself just as you are. If you are focusing on what you do not like, such as your flaws, and creating a problem that you need to somehow solve, this may give you some initial motivation when you come to the point where you are so fed up with things that you have no choice other than to take action. But how has this strategy for change worked for you so far?

17

You may find most of the time you feel down on yourself. You lack energy, motivation and procrastinate to another time when you'll feel 'up to it'. The fact is that you are playing at a losing strategy which will not support you to make lasting, positive change.

In Cognitive Behavioral Therapy, the core principle is about understanding that your thoughts directly affect your feelings, which directly affects the way you behave. So, if you are thinking negative thoughts about yourself, you're probably going to feel down about yourself and then you're probably going to turn to food for comfort. Or you'll binge, restrict and deprive yourself as punishment. Then you'll feel guilty for doing so—starting the cycle all over again. EAT>GUILT>REPENT>REPEAT!

So what about love? Love for ourselves means that we recognize our worthiness to be loved. When we love something we take care of it. You may have also heard the saying that in order to love others, we must first love ourselves. It is true that you cannot give anybody anything that you do not already have. If you wanted to give someone a dozen eggs, you'd first have to have a dozen eggs to give, right?

If we withhold love for ourselves, we are deeming ourselves unworthy of love. This may be because you've experienced a lack of love in your life from parents, caregivers or another significant person(s). Consider this, what if you loved and accepted yourself right now in this moment? Just play with the idea of what that would mean if you could love and accept yourself just as you are. If you are struggling with this consideration there is good work to be done.

If you do love and accept yourself just as you are, then great! There's still always some room for improvement! So, how do we improve our relationship with ourselves? First we have to accept ourselves just as we are and you can do that now can't you? If you've not been able to do that yet, then just consider how you can begin with respecting yourself. Respecting your body means you will take care of it and meet its basic needs. It also means you will be as gentle with yourself as you are with other people.

In order to improve your relationship with yourself here are some strategies you can apply in your life right now. These strategies are tools to help you to reframe and redefine any negative experiences or limiting beliefs you hold about yourself (such as I'm not worthy) and clear the way for you to accept where you are right now. Clear and present and ready to move forward without the baggage of your emotional past. You may also refer to www. eatguiltrepentrepeat.com for the companion workbook and audio toolkit.

These strategies are about training the habitual mind. In his book *The Principles of Psychology,* Professor William James, a well-known teacher and writer said: "The great thing in all education is to make our nervous system our ally instead of our enemy. For this we must make automatic and habitual, as early as possible, as many useful actions as we can and carefully guard against growing into ways that are likely to be disadvantageous. In the acquisition of a new habit or in the leaving off of an old one, we must take care to launch ourselves with strong and decided initiative as possible and never suffer an exception to occur until the new habit is securely rooted."

STRAGEY 1:

Shift your thoughts. Remember our thoughts affect our feelings and that affects our behavior. So switching your thoughts from what you don't want to what you do want will make a huge difference in how you will feel and act.

So if there was a part of you that you could love and appreciate just as it is what would that part be? Consider this may not be something physical. You are more than your body and size. Who are you? What is your nature? How do others see you? What would they say that part is? Do you have any qualities you like? Are you kind? Loving? Caring? Loyal?

Whenever you find yourself focusing on what you don't want and what you don't like, switch it to what you do want, what you do like.

Consider this, if you identified qualities in yourself like being a good friend, caring, kind or something similar would you consider being unkind, mean, hateful, hurtful, berating or foul towards someone you loved and cared about? Why not? Think about how that would affect them. It would probably make them really upset, wouldn't it? They may feel really bad about themselves and they may react in anger, dismay, or start crying, right? **SO WHY DO YOU THINK IT'S ACCEPTABLE FOR YOU TO TREAT YOURSELF IN THIS WAY?**

Jenny, now 43 had spent most of her life struggling to lose weight. She felt she could not consider acceptance of herself, even if it was about taking responsibility because she was sixty pounds overweight. She hated the way her body looked and didn't understand that was part of her problem. When I suggested her weight was a symptom of a deeper issue connected to her self-loathing she looked surprised. I asked her when she decided her body wasn't worthy of love and she couldn't remember a specific time. She had hated her body for so long that it seemed normal.

Using hypnosis we worked together to regress her back to the first time she felt this way towards herself. In trance, she remembered being bullied at school by an older group of girls. They picked on her and terrorized her. She remembered that she didn't understand why they hated her so much. She made a decision about herself at that time that it must be because she was fat and ugly. Jenny saw herself in a whole new way and formed a limiting belief based upon this significant emotional experience. This limiting belief imprinted on her mind was referred to time and time again as she continued to bully herself just as she had been bullied by others. Now Jenny was the biggest bully in her life.

Limiting beliefs shape our experience of reality. Another client, Carrie was bullied at school too. From the age of

8 she was taunted and teased by schoolmates about her size. She was taller and bigger although a normal, healthy weight for her frame. Her experience led to social withdrawal and as she became more isolated, she lost confidence in and around groups of people. Her lack of confidence was internalized and she developed a poor self-image about herself. Embarrassed about her body, she felt different from everyone else. This led to a limiting belief, "I am not good enough." When she looked in the mirror, she would call herself a "fat cow" and tell herself she was as "huge as a whale." Now 36 years old, the biggest bully in Carrie's life was her.

Like a long suffering victim of abuse, both Jenny and Carrie were comfortable and desensitized to the abuse at some level. Thoughts are real things to the mind. Even thoughts you've thought a hundred times, still on some level become things. In the case of the long-suffering victim, it perhaps reinforces a limiting belief, such as: "I am worthless", by providing yet more evidence that it is true.

It's more than just thinking positively about yourself. Thoughts are real things to the mind and they are instructions for how to feel and act. Everything you think is an affirmation. Whether it's something you want or don't like you are affirming this to yourself. Two of the most powerful words we use are I AM. The things you think or say to yourself about yourself framed as an identity statement become limiting beliefs. Beliefs are always true to the believer. They shape our perceptions of reality.

Worry is the child of fear. When we worry about things it's like praying for everything you do not want. Think of your thoughts as currency that buys all the things you want (or don't want) in your life. The best way to get rid of darkness is to let in the light. It is a waste of time to fight against a negative thought. You cannot deny it out of existence. The sheer denial of thought becomes a thought you hold in your mind. The best, surest and quickest method is to hold within your mind the desired outcome.

Instead of repeating "I am not afraid," say with conviction "I am full of courage," held firmly within the mind and with an attitude of courage, you will think it, feel it and begin to act on it. If you want to feel "good enough" then it is "I am deserving of good things," held firmly within the mind and with an attitude of worthy, you will think it, feel it and begin to act on it. The happiness you experience in your life depends on the quality of your thoughts.

Emotion is energy in motion. Habit is not divorced from feelings or emotion. In the very action of acquiring habits emotions deepen by repetition. If a person allows a feeling to take possession, the feeling becomes second nature to them. If this is undesirable emotion then only repetition of a more firmly entrenched emotion can rid or replace it.

So the problem isn't that you don't have the ability to create results. You are already doing that, but you are creating the results you do not want. Your mind, up to now, has been running on autopilot; unintentionally creating results. Once you take charge of how you focus your mind, and consciously and intentionally focus the spotlight of your mind on the outcome you want, you will find a way to make it happen in reality. I have never seen this fail.

This means that you have total control over your life. The only thing you can do to sabotage yourself is to allow your mind to run around loose, focusing unintentionally on what you are afraid of, what you don't want, what you don't like or what you want to avoid.

It is the 'blue tree syndrome'—don't think about a blue tree (*or anythingelse you don't want!*) I bet you thought about a blue tree. Well stop thinking of blue trees!!!!

Now stop thinking of pizza! See what happens? The mind thinks in images and representations of things. This means that when you try to stop or not think of something you are thinking of it. THOUGHTS = FEELINGS = ACTIONS.

So what do you want to think about instead? Here are some examples of what people typically say when they think of what they want:

"I don't want to be fat anymore"

"I don't want to overeat"

"I don't want to feel tired all the time"

"I don't want to be stressed out"

Make a list of what you want. Did you write what you didn't want and think this is what you want? Now what do you really want?! Go back through your list and refine your wants to ensure you are focusing on what you do want. When you catch yourself thinking and focussing on all the things you don't like or don't want, then **THINK AGAIN**. Use this as an alert or alarm bell to practice a new way of thinking of yourself.

"I don't want to be fat anymore" becomes "I am a healthy, natural weight."

"I don't want to overeat" becomes "I am eating the right amount to feel satisfied."

"I don't want to feel tired all the time" becomes "I am full of energy and motivation."

"I don't want to be stressed out" becomes "I am relaxed and at ease in any situation."

Whenever you find yourself thinking about the things you don't want—which is normal and inevitable, just say to yourself *"I know that's what I don't want, what do I want instead?"*

When you bring awareness in, you are no longer running on autopilot, you have a choice. The more you practice doing awareness, the more you will become awareness. All unresourceful thoughts fall by the wayside and are not even entertained.

STRATEGY 2:

Some people have that inner critic voice in their head that is always being harsh and saying things such as:

"I am so stupid"	"I know everyone thinks I'm fat"	"I am disgusting"
"I am fat and ugly"	"I am not good enough"	"I look awful"

These are thoughts in auditory form. Some people's inner critics are so engrained in their minds that they never think to challenge them. Everyone has inner dialogue; some have it more than others. Often, the voice takes on characteristics of other critical people we've come across in our life. Sometimes, we've just learned that this is the way we treat ourselves based on treatment we've experienced from others. We inherit and adopt our inner critic, but you do not have to let them live rent free in your mind. Negative self talk can be challenged and changed by redubbing the sound. So, what does that mean?

Your inner critic, or you can call it the 'storyteller', has a certain strategy for delivering their message. The way things sound affects us. So by changing the sound and qualities of the voice, you change your response to it. Your inner critic will talk to you in a certain tone, pitch and intensity. If you have one of these storytellers that speaks to you pay attention to the delivery. Notice how it sounds when it is saying negative, cruel things. Now I want you to imagine rewinding this and playing it back in the most silly and absurd voice you can imagine—such as Goofy, Donald Duck, Sponge Bob, Homer Simpson! Or imagine your own voice (or whosever voice it sounds like) with a high pitched helium effect.

Every time you catch the inner critic telling you stories you can use this as an alarm or alert to practice a new way of talking to yourself. You will need to make the effort to rewind and redub to make this effective. The point is a lot of what you say to yourself isn't true. It's just negative habitual thinking patterns that you're so accustomed to hearing you never thought to challenge. Every time you apply this strategy the storyteller gets weaker and becomes less effective at delivering their message. You find you just cannot take what the voice says seriously anymore and you can't can you? It may even make you smile.

When all else fails think of pink elephants because they are cute. Or ask yourself, what would a pink elephant say right now? Pink elephants are rarely abusive, unless they are drunk like in Disney's *Fantasia,* and this irreverent bit of writing is really to demonstrate that you have a choice to think and hear what you want. Also, pink elephants will most likely have a neutral association to them and will not trigger off a strong emotional reaction leading to limiting behaviors and results you do not want. If pink elephants do not work for you choose something else. Think again. It's your mind—you can use it however you want. Think whatever you want. It is your choice.

Another way you can change your storyteller is to focus on your immediate surroundings. Just check-in with what you notice around you. What do you see, hear, feel and what is the temperature of your environment in this moment? For example, you are standing in a room full of other people, you begin to compare yourself to others and your inner critic begins to tell you things which begin to impact you in a negative way such as, "I'm the fattest person in the room," or "Look, she's skinnier than me." Use this as an alarm bell to practice a new way of thinking and speaking to yourself!

"I see light blue curtains, the temperature is a bit warm, the glass I'm holding feels cold on my fingertips, my shoes feel tight, I'm fidgeting." This gives you present moment awareness.

AWARENESS IS KEY. The important thing is that you do this free of judgement. It should be neutral emotionally, which means you observe with non-judgemental awareness of the facts of the situation. If you find yourself still comparing and judging, then remember pink elephants!

Thoughts are real things to the mind and that includes auditory thoughts, but if you couldn't take them seriously, then they wouldn't affect you in the same way they did before and you don't need them to anymore—do you? Remember, you do not have to believe everything you think. If it isn't resourceful **THINK AGAIN**.

All it takes is practice. The more you do it, the easier it gets and in time the storyteller's voice changes permanently, so you never have to believe it ever again.

STRATEGY 3:

Have you ever heard of the Stop, Drop & Roll technique? It is a simple fire safety technique taught during health and safety training. A similar practice was developed by a psychologist and author Elisha Goldstein, PhD who deals in stress, anxiety and depression called S.T.O.P.

S—Stop whatever you are doing

T—Take a few deep breaths and notice the breath as it is, not trying to control the breath just using your breath as an anchor for this present moment

O—Observe your experience—what's happening in this moment in your mind, body and surroundings

P—Proceed by asking yourself, "What is most important to pay attention to right now?"

This strategy can be used with all the other strategies to help you cultivate awareness and be mindful of your thoughts, feelings and behaviors. The purpose of this strategy is to connect with the present moment fully to give you space of empowerment of choice and in this space between stimulus and response, connect with the inner wisdom within you.

To begin with you may want to keep yourself external reminders such as a post-it note with big words STOP or a picture of a stop sign to remind you. In order to get into routine, you'll at first need reminders to remember to do it! It only takes practice and practice makes permanent.

STRATEGY 4:

We all look in the mirror every day, but rarely do we make eye contact with ourselves when we do. You're brushing your hair, teeth, applying make-up or even looking in the rear view mirror of your car, but never actually looking directly at yourself. If you do manage to look at yourself, you are probably looking at all the things you hate, dislike, want to change, that are missing or you see the lack.

Mirror work involves making a conscious effort to change this. When you do look in the mirror and you remember to do so, make direct eye contact with yourself and say something nice. I recommend the following, **"I love and accept myself just as I am."**

Don't worry if you don't believe it (yet), that they are just words or that it's difficult for you to do. Let that be just a part of the process of change. The belief will follow the repetition as you begin to feel more positive and nurturing towards yourself by applying these strategies into your day-to-day-routine.

If you find this too difficult then start with **"I am willing to learn to like myself" or "I am respecting my body and thank it for supporting me"** and go from there.

STRATEGY 5:

You may want to consider writing a letter of apology to your younger self. This could be written to the younger you at that time you made a decision about yourself that is related to a poor relationship to yourself now.

Both Jenny and Carrie wrote a letter to their younger selves. Jenny has shared hers.

Dear little Jenny,

I made it really hard for you to feel good about yourself. I mistreated you and for that I am deeply sorry. All you wanted was to feel good and be happy, but I hurt you and put you down. When I should have taken care of you, I ignored your needs. I turned to food for comfort and put toxins in you which affected your health. I feel terrible because I know that yourself esteem was in the dumpster and this affected how you let others treat you. All you wanted was to be loved and I didn't love you.

You sought love and acceptance from others and you were let down and this only made you believe it was true that you were unlovable. I am sorry I shamed you and called you nasty names. I didn't make you feel safe or worthy of good things and that you mattered. I know you wanted desperately to please others so they would love you and accept you.

I realize now that this was not possible because you didn't love and accept yourself. I am writing you today and from the bottom of my heart I ask you for your forgiveness. I love you. You are beautiful. Please forgive me.

Thank you, Jenny

When Jenny brought this letter into our next session, she asked if I wanted to read it. I asked her to read it out loud. After she read the letter I asked her how she felt about it. She explained how tearful she was writing this letter and realized how much hurt was inside of her. She sat with this feeling and allowed her imagination to wander where she imagined comforting the little girl who then took her hand and wanted to play dolls with her. Afterwards, she said she felt lighter and whole again. I asked her how her younger self was doing and she said she was fine and off doing things that little girls should be doing.

Jenny had made peace with herself and began with healing her current relationship with her body. It was interesting as Jenny not only seemed happier and lighter, she looked it too. Our emotional baggage is a weight we carry. When you shed the emotional baggage, you literally lighten up.

Our unconscious image of ourselves is who we believe we are and this is the end result of everything we have learned and programmed in our minds. The process of transformation is about becoming aware, recognizing, identifying and updating the programs by deleting old programmes and installing new ones. All our limitations come from unresolved issues and limiting beliefs we hold. We are only limited by our limitation of what we believe is possible. What you believe is a product of parents, peers, teachers and others who have helped you to form an idea of who you are. If you believe you are unlovable, not good enough, not deserving and not attractive then you are limiting yourself to a lower level experience of reality. You have forgotten who you really are as an unlimited being of love buried beneath years of conditioning.

STRATEGY 6:

Befriending ourselves is really a process of acceptance and integration. The part of you that you do not like, that you want to hide from the world, that you feel is unacceptable is the best part of you. That may be hard to understand, but by integrating this part of you, you are becoming whole again.

Victoria was certain that she could not accept herself as she was. She was adamant that it was impossible for her to love her body just as it was. To her, she was ugly and only when she had lost weight and returned to her former size, would she be able to feel good about her body. For years, she had struggled with her body image. When she walked through town she felt as though all eyes were on her. Everyone was judging her for being overweight.

Her long-term relationship ended as her boyfriend rejected her because she was ugly and fat. She was so insecure and jealous and she didn't trust him. She was convinced he had cheated on her with her friends. Not only did she lose her relationship with this man, she lost her friendship too.

Her life was a mess. She had let herself go completely.

She didn't care about her health and ate her feelings. She wallowed in self pity every night. Her only solace was when she was at work. At work, she could throw herself into it and forget she felt so worthless and insecure. In her high powered position, she spent a lot of time proving to others how important she was. She garnered the respect of others by acting bulletproof. She admitted it was only an act. Inside she felt like she was weak and insecure but at work she felt like a tough gal. It made her feel good, if only temporarily. Every evening, when she returned home and she was left with nothing but her own company, she was thrown into despair. She would in her words, "turn into a food zombie" who ate in order to fill the gap and escape her pain.

Her behavior was becoming more and more unstable. She felt as though she was losing the plot and heading for a nervous

Brenda J. Bentley

breakdown. Not only was she eating her feelings, she began drinking too much.

"When I drink, I feel more confident. I go out to my local bar and after a few drinks, I am able to talk to and flirt with people. I really love the attention I get from others. The next day, I feel awful. I have a headache and I've even started drinking in the mornings to try to get over my hangover. I really feel as though I am self destructing."

One evening she went out to a local club she hadn't been before. She had already been drinking at home, but wanted to get out of the house where she knew she would end up eating her night away again. After a few drinks she struck up conversation with some guys at the bar. They bought her drinks and they played a few games of pool. One of the guys was flirting with her and she enjoyed the attention. The night wore on and after too many drinks, she decided it was time to call a taxi to get home. She announced her intention to leave, but the guys were asking her to stay. She stayed for another drink, after all, what did she have to look forward to at home?

At some point, she can't recall, she realized that she wasn't feeling herself. She felt woozy and out of sorts. She asked her new friends to help her and the last thing she remembers is being pushed into a taxi accompanied by one of the guys.

The next day, she awoke in bed naked, she was alone in an apartment and she had no idea how she had got there. Her head was bursting and she looked for her clothes. She found them and got dressed and went into the kitchen. There wasn't anyone home. No signs of the guys she met the night before. She checked and she had all of her belongings and felt relieved. She called a taxi and went home.

When she got home, she realized that something had to change. Her experience was a wake-up call. How could she not even remember what happened? Was she drugged? Did she have sex with that guy? There was no way to know the truth. She resolved at that point to get help and that's when she contacted me. She didn't want to end up dead one day because of her irresponsible behaviors.

As she told me her story I could see how she was motivated to make a change. When I asked her what she wanted she said that she wanted to be happy. If she lost weight, she'd be more confident and that would mean she could be happy again.

She'd be able to attract a man who she could have a loving relationship with. He would love her because she was slim and beautiful. This would mean she wouldn't be desperate for the attention of others or feel lonely any longer. It would also mean she wouldn't be jealous because everyone would be envious of her. Her only hope was to lose weight and she wanted me to fix her.

During our sessions she rejected everything about learning the strategies. Everything I offered her to consider was dismissed. I threw my hands up, "You know, you're right. There is no use in trying to convince you otherwise. In fact, I think we should consider that the work we've done here is finished."

With that Victoria looked shocked. She immediately dropped the tough gal act and looked wounded.

"I don't know what else to do," she wept.

I told Victoria that I am teaching her exactly what she needs to do, but she doesn't want to even consider doing it. In order to be free you need to make whole that which you have rejected.

This means you need to integrate the part of you that you have dismissed as being unworthy, ugly and unlovable.

Victoria looked me directly in the eye and for the first time I heard her open up and she asked, "How do I do that?"

Insecurity creates a barrier between us and other people. We push other people away as we believe we do not have the qualities inside that are worthy of genuine love. When we are insecure we are preoccupied with how others perceive us. We are obsessed with the perception that other people are judging us in an unkind way. We are convinced that all of our flaws are plastered all over ourselves and we scramble in an attempt to hide them.

We interpret other people's comments and actions as being hurtful and untrustworthy. In fact, we are projecting all of our insecurities onto others becoming even more alienated and disconnected from others. What Victoria began to recognize is that she had become self centered. In her attempt to keep people from seeing the part of her that was vulnerable, she came off as abrasive and pompous. This caused other people to feel uneasy about her. She realized it wasn't other people who rejected her, she had pushed others away from her!

Insecurity cannot be remedied by obtaining high powered positions, money, academic degrees or by losing weight, you must integrate and make whole the parts of you so you no longer project them onto other people. No amount of validation, praise or recognition can eliminate the insecurity. You crave acceptance and search for this outside of yourself. You only need to look at some celebrities and their struggles to see that. Your quest for external validation means you hide all the aspects of yourself you fear others will not like. Your shadow self becomes the dumpster where all the things you do not accept about yourself are buried underneath your worst qualities. In doing so, the best part of yourself becomes something you despise.

Carl Jung was a Swiss psychologist and psychiatrist who founded analytical psychology and was the first person to refer to this part of us as the "shadow". The shadow is an archetype personality, which simply means it is a model of a person, personality or behavior. Jung believed that the shadow aspect of ourselves is an unconscious aspect of the personality which the conscious ego does not recognize in itself.

The shadow is an accumulation of all the repressed, suppressed or disowned qualities of the conscious self. According to Jung, people deal with their shadow in four ways: denial, projection, integration and/or transmutation. The shadow has both constructive and destructive aspects. Insecure people tend to dismiss their positive attributes and focus largely on their negative aspects.

"Everyone carries a shadow," Jung wrote, "and the less it is embodied in the individual's conscious life, the blacker and denser it is."

According to Jung, the shadow, in being instinctive and irrational, is prone to projection. It turns a perceived inferiority into real deficiency in someone else. If the projections are unrecognized the shadow has free reign to cripple the person as the foggy illusion forms between egocentric self and reality.

Inside of all of us is this shadow self that we are deeply ashamed of. No matter how hard you try you cannot escape this shadow. You cannot get rid of this part of you. It is called the shadow because it follows you everywhere. The only time you are free from your shadow is when you bring it into the light and see it for what it is.

Brenda J. Bentley

Integration of the Shadow Self

Integration is done with a powerful exercise using your imagination. Remember a time when you felt insecure and recreate the feelings you had. Imagine you can push those feelings out in front of you so they take form as a person with a face and body. This is the personification of your insecurity. This is your shadow self. It doesn't matter how this is being represented. It may even change during the process of your transformation. This shadow represents everything you do not want to be, but fear you are.

As you become familiar with this part of you, imagine that you can form an indestructible bond between you and your shadow. You may want to imagine this as a cord of light, like an imaginary umbilical cord that you can siphon the strengths and resources of your shadow. As you face your shadow, respecting this bond between you, acknowledge, accept, show appreciation and thank this part of you for being here. Notice how this changes everything. Now with this part of you united and working in partnership in complete agreement you can turn and face your day or any challenge with a new found confidence.

Using this strategy you can breakthrough and integrate all insecurities and come to a place of peaceful contentment for who you really are. You may need to repeat this often and notice how every time you do this, if the shadow self changes in representation.

To others Victoria was a strong, capable executive whose confidence came across as arrogance. To herself, she was an ugly, grotesque, fat monster of a person who was unworthy of good things. After integration, Victoria is much more peaceful, her shadow self has transformed to a purer reflection of herself.

I have experienced and my clients have shared how their shadow self changes each time they integrate. The high powered executive's shadow changes from a weak, vulnerable little girl hiding her face to a young woman who is standing upright and displays confidence. The college professor whose shadow was a gnarled and twisted creature changed to a robust and handsome medal-worthy athlete. We can both wonder how your shadow self will transform with practice.

The secret to transforming your life is not in reading this book. Transformation is in experiencing this book by applying yourself to learn and use its tools and strategies. It may even take a few weeks before you begin to notice and experience real change in your life. Be realistic in your expectations and remember the most important thing is that you take action and apply these strategies into your life. Consider these teachings like a seed I'm giving to you. You can take these seeds and disregard them or you could plant them, nurture them and watch them grow. In this instance, by applying them into your day-to-day, moment-by-moment life and nurturing yourself with kind thoughts, which will lead to kind feelings—you can just imagine how much better you will feel already, can't you?

Improving your relationships takes the time it takes for you to begin to feel and know it's different. Change is a process, not a destination. How fast change happens will depend on how deeply engrained the old ways of thinking, feeling and acting is.

Remember, a habit is just something that you do over and over again. Certainly, this way is a much more positive and powerful habit to have that will change your life forever in every area. Make the effort and do the work it takes—you'll only feel great about yourself.

This is the basis of changing your relationship with yourself, but in further chapters there will be additional insight and action steps for you to hone what you're learning, bringing this into experiential knowledge.

Action Steps:

1. Ask yourself what you really want in your life.

2. Make a list of what you want based on your solution state.

3. Consider acceptance and gift yourself with empowerment.

4. Practice a new way of thinking with strategies continuously.

5. Practice mirror work. Say it like you mean it and commit yourself to make it true.

6. Write a heartfelt letter of forgiveness to yourself and make peace.

7. Continue to nurture yourself with love, kindness and self compassion.

8. Integrate your shadow aspects.

9. Repeat!

Chapter 3—Food is Your Friend

"Hunger: One of the few cravings that cannot be appeased with another solution."
~ Irwin Van Grove

We learn immediately at birth that food is comforting. Babies cry out for feeding and when this is responded to appropriately their hunger and satiety signals are reinforced. Try to get a baby to eat when they are not hungry and what happens? A lot of nothing happens! A baby will not eat when they are not hungry and will stop when they have finished, and this happens many times throughout the day and night as they are in tune with their instinctive signals of hunger and satiety.

This relationship changes as we grow up through conditioning from our environment and caregivers as they influence how and when we eat. Our eating becomes structured, practical and based on timing and other external stimulus and less on our own bodies. There are those who have maintained their instinctual relationship with food despite outside influences.

What is your relationship with food?

Good. I eat when I'm hungry and have a balanced diet.

Varied. Sometimes good, sometimes not so good.

Bad. I eat lots of junk food, more than I should for the wrong reasons.

What are your eating habits like?

Eat only when hungry

Brenda J. Bentley

Stop when satisfied

Eat a varied diet including fresh fruit & veg

Eat when alone

Eat in secret

Feel guilty after eating

Eat all the time

Constantly think about food

Eat certain types of foods more than others

Eat certain times of day more than others

Don't pay attention to any of this

Eat when doing other things like watching TV or surfing the 'net'

Eating is a way to escape my problems

Eating is a way to comfort myself

Eating is a way to reward myself

Eating by rules is a way I feel more in control.

Eating until I'm full up is a way I feel safe.

If you've checked any boxes besides eat only when hungry, stop when satisfied, eat a varied diet then there is improvement to be made with your relationship with food.

Food has many different roles and purposes in our lives. When we find ourselves with an unhealthy relationship, we need to look to our past to explore any potential link to our present attitudes and relationship with food. We learn how to have a poor relationship with food through imitation or modelling the behavior of others, mostly through those who are in a position of influence—parents, caregivers and siblings. We inherit limiting beliefs and values about food, such as 'having to finish everything on your plate' or as I refer to this outdated value system 'clean plate syndrome'.

When we are young our minds are developing and we are in our formative stages neurologically. These stages can be defined as: the imprint period, from birth to about age 7 years old, the modelling period from 7-14 years old, and the socialisation period, from about 14-21 years old.

During the imprint period, up to age 7, our minds have only a few ways to filter information as it comes in through your senses. Think about the innocence of a child or how a child's mind is like a sponge. This means you become imprinted very easily as you do not have the same capacity to block certain types of input as an adult would.

In the modelling period, from 7-14 years old, the child makes choices about who to model. This is the period of hero-worship, where kids idolize Harry Potter, sports figures, parents, TV and movie stars, rock stars, older brothers or sisters, the more popular of their peers, and so on, and then adopt parts of their values from these heroes.

In the socialisation period, from ages 14-21, the young adult begins to adopt social, sexual and personal values and is less likely to adopt something just because someone else is doing it.

In the imprint stages, safety is the essential directive used by the unconscious mind in choosing what to adopt. The unconscious part of our minds is governed by this directive of safety and protection. This means that beliefs and attitudes of others observed will become hardwired as synaptic pathways in the unconscious mind. Young children carefully observe then download information offered by parents and caregivers directly into their unconscious minds. Why is this important to know? So you can understand how and when you came to develop your poor relationship with food and how to unlearn and grow out of this and into a healthy and resourceful relationship with food.

So what role did food play in your life as a child?

When we examine our historical relationship with food we can begin to gain insight into where and how our eating patterns were influenced and learned.

Was eating regular and routine?

Were there certain times to eat?

Was there enough for everyone?

Were you made to finish everything on your plate?

If so, was this a negative emotional experience for you?

Was food ever used as a form of punishment? Example: sent to bed without dinner.

Was there competitive eating between you and others?

Did you ever feel deprived?

Were you envious of what others were allowed and you were not?

Was food used as a reward when you were good?

Was food given to you to comfort you when you were upset?

Were you aware of either of your parents' dieting behaviors?

If yes, then how did this affect you?

When did you first begin to struggle with your weight?

If it was during your childhood—what was going on at the time?

We have emotional and psychological needs that need to be met throughout our life. If these are not met, then we find a means to an end to have them satisfied, and food can be one of those means we learn to use.

If food gave you something beyond nutrition and sustenance what would you say?

Food is

Remember you are looking to discover things that are giving you the most negative result. Don't write in what you *think it should mean*, but what it does mean to you. For example:

Food is <u>a way that I deal with stress</u>

Be honest with yourself. When you are able to identify your underlying relationship you can clear the way for healthier patterns of behavior. Is there an emotional or psychological need that food is meeting for you? Perhaps you are using food to deal with uncomfortable emotions.

Helen was one of six children in a big Catholic family. She was the youngest girl with two older sisters, two older brothers and one younger brother. Food was the centerpiece of their daily family interaction. They ate and sat at the table together for breakfast of porridge and toast. Lunch at school was a packed lunch of the ordinary childhood lunch staples and sandwiches. The evening meal was shared again with classic home cooked dinners made by her mother. She was raised in a very disciplined way. She had chores and table manners were really important. She was taught the right way to hold a fork and knife, napkin on her lap, and she wouldn't eat and drink at the same time for fear of a slap to her head from one of her parents skilfully observing and 'teaching' proper behavior. She also learned that food must never be wasted. In a large family, although they had plenty, you always ate everything that was given to you. Each child got the same amount regardless of age, appetite or preference. She learned to eat things she didn't like, like brussels sprouts and cauliflower.

One night, she was given liver and onions and although she tried to eat everything, she found herself retching whenever she attempted to put the liver anywhere close to her mouth. This was observed and noted by her dutiful parents, who assured her that she would not be leaving the table until every last mouthful was eaten. She settled in for the long haul. She sat there just short of four hours before she was excused from the table thinking she'd won this power struggle, only to find liver and onions on her breakfast plate the next morning. When it wasn't eaten then, she had it in-between two slices of her bread for lunch . . . of which she put in the garbage at school and hoped no one would notice. Unfortunately, her parents' eyes had seen through her scheme as her older sister tattled. She was punished with no dinner that night and made to do extra chores as penance.

You can understand based on Helen's story how her relationship with food became contaminated. Her emotional and psychological connection to food was that of discipline, structure, obedience and conformity. It's not wrong to learn good manners or to not to waste food, but for Helen, food became the enemy. She developed a rebellious attitude towards foods she 'should eat' and as an adult rebelled against herself and others who tried to tell her otherwise.

"When my husband wasn't around, I would eat anything I wanted, mostly cakes and candy bars until I felt sick. I looked forward to him leaving so I could do so without his judgemental stares."

Helen also learned that she had to get the food she wanted quickly as it was a highly competitive environment with her siblings. Her parents controlled the amount of sugar and sweets they could have which became a powerful bartering tool. This meant that when Helen had grown-up, sugary foods were what she wanted the most and she learned to sneak and hide them from others in her family, specifically, her children, so she could have them when she was alone.

"I remember putting pop-tarts in the back of the cupboard behind the old can of peaches so no one would find them, it was my secret stash, just ready and waiting for me." She also had very little satisfaction when eating these foods, except for the fleeting feeling of power it gave her.

So she was eating foods she didn't really want, when she didn't really want them, based on ticking an emotional / psychological box in her head which she wasn't even aware existed. She was setting rules for herself based on her parents structured and disciplined way of behaving and subsequently was passing these same lessons on to her own children. These value judgements are inherited and then passed along from generation to generation without critical analysis of whether or not they are helpful or hurtful.

What is your story? What lessons were you taught? Did you inherit any value judgements about wasting food? By examining your historical and current relationship with food and what you do consistently, you can begin to identify these connections to the moods that accompany your urge to eat. If you ate when you were hungry and only when you were hungry, and you could eat whatever you wanted, not what you thought you should or when you thought you should, and stopped when you were satisfied you would not struggle with your weight. Your body would naturally find its default healthy weight that is right for you—*effortlessly*.

Eat what you want—**WHEN YOU ARE HUNGRY**

Not what you think you should—**THERE ARE NO GOOD AND BAD FOODS**

Not when you think you should—**JUST BECAUSE IT'S LUNCH TIME DOESN'T MEAN YOU EAT**

STOP WHEN YOU ARE SATISIFIED—Satisfaction does not mean **FULLNESS**

Hunger is your body's way of telling you it is time to eat.

It's part of your primitive, instinctual, reactive response.

It's about sustaining life, keeping you healthy and well. So how come most people eat when they are not hungry because it is lunchtime or dinnertime even though they are not hungry? Conditioning—they have learned to do this.

If you eat when you are not hungry it is like stopping and getting fuel for your vehicle when it doesn't need it. You wouldn't stop to fill up your car when it didn't require more fuel would you? Can you imagine if you had to use the toilet based on a schedule and telling yourself, "No, I'm going to ignore this signal to urinate and follow a schedule which rules when I can relieve my bladder."

It sounds crazy that you would provide fuel when it wasn't necessary or create strict rules to follow in an attempt to control your natural urges, doesn't it? You can learn a different way of eating food which works and honours your body and its needs so you can return to the healthy, natural, default weight that is right for you. Re-training your mind to know the difference between genuine hunger and emotional hunger just takes awareness and practice. What is a habit after all? It's a behavior that you repeat over and over again until it becomes automatic—second nature.

To change the underlying reason for your problem, you have worked to identify the *key area* where your problem resides. Is it a poor relationship with yourself? A poor relationship with food? Perhaps it is both. Trust your findings and go with your intuition.

Think of your behaviors as symptoms of these poor relationships which means your thoughts and your feelings are at the core of processing this change. If we change your thoughts you will feel differently and you will subsequently behave differently. You can do this by changing or unlearning the learned behaviors you've discovered.

At this point a lot of people become sceptical. They do not trust themselves to eat whatever they want. The trust in themselves has eroded with each failed attempt to lose weight. It is understandable why you would feel this way. In order to heal your relationship with food, you need to make peace with it. Consider that if you were able to eat whatever you want, you wouldn't feel deprived. It is only at this point when you are **FREE** to make choices that supportive choice can be made.

You may find yourself totally freaking out right now and running to the cupboard to binge on all those forbidden foods you've denied yourself. You may not trust yourself enough to even know what hunger feels like. You may have ignored hunger for so long that it's become normal for you. There may be a lot of conflicting messages you will hear out in the world that will tell you that it's insane to approach food like this. The only thing you need to do right now is consider that if you were to allow yourself to eat whatever you wanted with the only stipulation that you were hungry could you allow yourself to learn about yourself?

This process is about learning about yourself. You are the expert of yourself. No one else can know you better than you do. You, however have turned outside of yourself to find the answers that are inherent, but latent inside of you. Right now, you may not be able to reference this inner strength and wisdom, but as you read this book you are being given the tools to peer inside of yourself to explore and discover your greatest truths.

These truths have been buried inside under years of conditioning. Your job is to take action to peel back each layer and expose the truth that lies beneath. It may sound daunting and complicated. I assure you it is not. It only takes courage and willingness to consider and you've already done that. Take a moment to appreciate that about yourself. You are willing to consider change.

Action Steps:

1. Consider your relationship with food

2. What is your story?

3. What lessons were you taught?

4. What values did you inherit?

5. What is your key for transformation? Food or yourself? Perhaps it is both?

6. Be open to learning more about yourself.

Chapter 4—Imagination: The Tool for Transformation

"If my mind can conceive it, and my heart can believe it, I know I can achieve it."
~ Jesse Jackson, American Civil Rights Leader

So let's now introduce the process by which change happens: Using your imagination in a powerful and positive way. Albert Einstein said, "Imagination is a preview of life's coming attractions." This is because the core of transformation is all about your thoughts—and thoughts are real things to the mind. They really affect you either negatively or positively. Sometimes it seems as though there's no effect because we aren't really thinking of anything at all or we are unaware of what we are thinking. This is when we are engaged fully in the present moment activity, which is rarely experienced as a thought.

Thoughts are about thinking, reviewing, analyzing, planning, problem solving, rationalizing and even daydreaming. Most of the time your process of thinking happens automatically, unintentionally and beneath your conscious awareness. Your mind thinks thoughts, you experience thoughts, perhaps you are aware of the thoughts, thinking the thoughts, as they come and go in and out of your awareness. Or perhaps you are thinking you do experience your thoughts in solving problems, answering questions, crossword puzzles and other such activities. This is purposeful thinking and rarely produces problems in, and of, itself, except when allowed to wander through worst case scenarios or fear-based agendas.

You are probably thinking right now *what is this all about?*

Thinking is part of your conscious mind. When you are awake, you primarily are in your conscious mind—this means what you are aware of and how you engage with the world through your senses. It is everything you see, hear, taste, touch, smell and know (thoughts you are aware of) at any given moment. It is your cognitions. It is your mental processes and functions, your attention, understanding and processing language and problem solving. It is the rational, logical, analytical and reasoning part of your thinking processes. It is also your short-term memory and your moment-to-moment decision making facility.

When you are awake you are using your conscious mind, your cognitive facilities to make sense of the world around you. To take in stimulus through your senses and to make decisions based on the information you've taken in. Some of these decisions happen automatically or unconsciously—and I will cover that in a moment. So the decisions such as: "Do I want coffee or tea?", "Do I want a cookie or a banana?", "Do I want to turn left or right at the next junction?" are all made with your conscious mind with your decision making facility.

Most diets are run using the conscious mind. This is why diets seem like so much work. Using mental energy to make decisions and choose the banana over the cookie is an effort. This is why you can do diets for short-term success, but after awhile, you fall back upon the learned behaviors when you no longer have the energy to continue to make the choices you *should* be making to follow a diet.

Relying on the conscious mind to do this not only takes effort, but it is as if you are talking to the doorman of an apartment building, asking and trying to purchase the building from them. The point is you need to get the source, root cause of the concern. This is the learned behavior which is driving the problem. This belongs to the unconscious mind.

The unconscious mind is sometimes referred to as the 'subconscious' mind. I refer to it as the 'unconscious' mind but we can refer to it as the 'automatic' mind. This means it is everything you do *automatically without having to think about it*.

Things like healing, digestion, blood flow, muscle movements, the way our hair and nails grow, the way your heart beats, blinking your eyes . . . You do not have to think about those things for them to happen do you. That is because they are all a responsibility of the unconscious mind.

Creating new behaviors and habits comes from the decision to learn a new way of doing things. Like when you learned to drive a car, you decided you wanted to learn how to do it, because you realized all the benefits and freedom that learning this would bring you. Or if you don't drive, then think about tying your shoes.

When I was younger, I watched my mother in awe. She was able to talk on the phone, watch over dinner on the stove and tie my shoes before I was able to do it all at the same time! I was convinced my mother was a wizard with special powers. My immense struggle with learning this skill, over hours of concentrative stares with tongue sticking out ever so slightly, took what seemed years to come to fruition. It is kind of embarrassing to admit that, but it demonstrates the point. It meant a lot to me to learn how to tie my shoes; I wanted the freedom from having to run home for help whenever I inevitably found myself with strings undone and tripping over my laces.

The tenacity of this desire made me realize how this is very much like learning anything new. At first it seems like a lot of stuff to learn. Then, with practice, it becomes easier and easier and now, I'm proud to say, I can tie my shoes whilst multi-tasking as well! Wizards unite! A foolish brag? No. Anything you learn that is new takes practice. Walking, talking, riding a bike, playing an instrument and this. This will take the effort it takes to create a new automatic learned behavior and you start with your desire and decision to learn. Learned behaviors you do become the responsibility of the unconscious mind so they can be performed with little or no conscious mental energy expended.

Our minds do not know the difference between real things and imagined ones. What we think about can affect our physiological states. Your thoughts are real things to the mind. That is why you can think about something that was upsetting and get upset now. Worry, stress, anxiety are all products of our thoughts where we imagine things going the way we don't want them to in the future. This affects our present moment and can induce a fear-based response in the moment. The power of our mind affects our experience of life, which means we can use our imagination in a powerful and positive way to create the desired change. In doing so, you can use your mind to accelerate the learning process, create new thoughts, feelings and behaviors that support transformation.

Our conscious and unconscious minds work together seamlessly in tandem with each other. The unconscious mind takes over the moment your conscious mind is not paying attention and is responsible for your autonomy. Your conscious mind can travel through time—to the past and into the future whilst the unconscious mind is infinite and timeless or always in the present moment (no time). So while your mind is thinking, wandering, analyzing, planning, reviewing, your unconscious mind can just get on with what it needs to without the need for supervision.

The Language of the Unconscious Mind

Now you understand the two different parts of the mind and their responsibilities, it's important to understand the process of learning or reprogramming your mind. Hypnosis is a powerful

53

tool that you can use to make changes at an unconscious level. It's a safe, natural and effective means to create changes using the imagination in a powerful and positive way. Hypnosis has a long and colourful history dating back to the times of the Egyptians. There are a lot of myths and misconceptions about hypnosis and what it is capable of doing. The most important thing you need to understand is that hypnosis is a natural state— it is not a special state induced by a hypnotist that pulls you into a trance and can control your mind and force you to do things you wouldn't want to do yourself.

It is not mind control. It is not magic. It is a safe, natural and effective means for using the language of the unconscious mind—and the means to do this is by engaging the imagination in a powerful and positive way. The unconscious mind is about pictures, images, symbolism, metaphors, dreams and emotion. It does not distinguish between good and bad, right and wrong— its only directive is safety and protection and it will reject anything that would threaten that.

Also your conscious mind, acting as a gatekeeper is a filter which will reject anything which doesn't agree with your ideas, values and beliefs that you hold for yourself. You are always in control. You cannot stay in hypnosis. Humans go in and out of a hypnosis-like state throughout the day. Think of hypnosis as a 'focussed state of concentration'—whenever you are focussed on something like driving a car, reading an interesting book or watching a good film, you are focussed and not aware of all the things going on around you. This in essence is what hypnosis is. It's concentrating on something so you miss the details of other things going on around you. That is why when you are driving a routine journey, you don't even think about it; you arrive at your destination and don't even remember driving there!

Available to you is a free self hypnosis audio recording you can download from www.eatguiltrepentrepeat.com to guide and accelerate the change you desire for yourself. In order to unlearn learned behaviors which are the responsibility of the unconscious mind, you need to go to the source. Whether this learning happened by inheritance, modelling, imprinting, conditioning or repetition—it all belongs to you and is accessible by working with how your mind stores information. Also by understanding your mind you create a space for choice so you are no longer running on auto-pilot, giving yourself the empowerment of choice.

The reason I refer to this part of your mind as unconscious in lieu of sub-conscious is that 'sub' suggests that it is existing or operating beneath the surface and beyond reach. The modern view is that all hypnosis is self hypnosis. Hypnosis provides us with a way to fast track change as we are working with the root cause of the problem and the source of the solution. This gives you an extraordinary way to empower yourself to tap into strengths, resources and abilities you may not have realized you have or that limiting beliefs you hold keep you from realizing. Using your imagination in a powerful and positive way acts like a primer to link your transformation to making your life more fun and interesting, so the more likely it is that you make this a long-term part of your lifestyle. Live these goals, think about them often, and *repeat*! Daydream about it, understand, know and feel how good it will feel to have this transformation realized. Your imagination is the most powerful and positive resource you have and it's free!

Your transformation begins with what you think.

Samantha was a 37 year old accountant, who came to see me to lose weight. During the intake consultation, she said she had been diagnosed with irritable bowel syndrome which caused a lot of discomfort for her. Her doctors told her that it could be stress related and gave her my contact details.

She told me she was working long hours at her job and wasn't very happy about that. She had even started working at the weekends. She felt she didn't have a life. She felt tired to the point where no amount of sleep helped. In fact, she couldn't sleep. Her sleep was interrupted with distressing thoughts about her not waking up on time to be the first in the office. It was affecting every area of her life. She was single and didn't have a social life. Her friends felt as though they didn't matter and rarely invited her out anymore. Work had become her life, but she was beginning to dread going to work. She felt she needed to work the extra time as she was being considered for a partner position within the firm. She felt a lot of pressure to prove herself and took on extra work but realized she was burning out in the process.

All of the emotion was concentrated right in her gut. She turned to food for comfort which contributed to her increasing weight. Her food choices also aggravated her IBS. The more stress she felt, the more her stomach knotted up. The more her stomach knotted up the more stress she felt.

When I asked her what she was afraid would happen if she worked a normal number of hours she explained how she felt she would be letting herself down. She also feared she would be overlooked when it came to the promotion. I asked if she believed that her boss would think less of her for having a healthy work and life balance and she answered, "No." She seemed surprised with the answer that came out of her mouth.

Do you think that your boss would appreciate it if you were working at your peak performance? What if you felt refreshed, eager, enthusiastic, happy and motivated at work? Do you think that would make a difference in considering you as the best candidate for the partnership?

It became clear to Samantha that she had been looking at things from a completely different angle and this is what needed to be changed. The realization alone helped, but she was still unsure how she was going to break the cycle.

Using Samantha's imagination we focussed on the feeling of stress she experienced and where she could feel it in her body. Not surprising, she felt it in her stomach. I had her focus intently on this feeling, giving herself permission to allow it to be present. I then asked her to imagine all the way back into her past when she felt this feeling the first time.

Samantha recalled when she younger, about 15 years old and she was in high school, she had a close friend in whom she trusted and confided all of her secrets. One of the secrets she told her friend was that she wanted to quit her athletics program at school to pursue cheerleading. She knew that her mother was not keen for her to pursue cheerleading and never allowed her or supported her in doing so in the past. She decided to do this on her own and went to the cheerleading tryouts and secured a place on the squad without the knowledge and permission of her parents. She had forged her mother's signature on the permission slip and paid for the dues for her uniform with her babysitting money. This friend betrayed her confidence and told her parents. When her parents discovered the truth, they confronted her at cheerleading practice. In front of everyone, she was humiliated as her dishonesty was exposed. When she confronted her friend about her betrayal, her friend told her that she didn't want to be friends any longer as she didn't want a liar as a friend. Her friend dumped her on the spot and she was devastated. Samantha felt ashamed and that she was no good and in fact a bad person with no redeeming qualities.

I asked her what the connection was between this event and the stress she experienced and she told me that it was the shame. She was afraid of people rejecting her because she was no good. When I asked what it was her younger self believed about herself as a result of the experience she said in a matter of fact style, "I am no good."

As a result of her having this belief she internalized her fear and set to please everyone around her even if this was at the expense of her health. Using Samantha's imagination, I asked her to allow her unconscious mind to absorb any learning, understandings or insights about the time that would be useful for her letting the limiting belief go completely and for good. It didn't actually matter if she knew what these things were, but just to imagine that there were some. Just to imagine that she could pass this insight to her younger self, using her imagination in a powerful and positive way, so that she could look at her younger self and know that she knows it now. She let me know when she had finished and to her surprise, she felt different. We tested and checked that the feeling had changed to neutral and allowed her to continue to use her imagination as I guided her to consolidate all the subsequent experiences she had where that limiting belief was present.

Afterwards, Samantha was asked to check where that feeling was she had when she started this exercise and she commented she couldn't get it back. She knew where it was before, but it didn't feel like it used to. I asked her what it is she believed about herself based on what the younger self had learned today and she replied, "I am a good person and I deserve balance."

From that point on Samantha recognized that in order to give others the best of her, she had to put herself first. Saying yes to someone else should never come at the cost to saying no to yourself. Putting yourself first is not selfish; it just means you care about others enough to give them your best. Your best means that you take care of yourself and live a healthy and balanced life.

This is one example of the power of your imagination to affect positive change. You can check the resources section of this book to find details of the accompanying workbook and additional audio recordings to support your transformation.

Chapter 5—Belief is the Foundation of Perception

"If you believe you can or you believe you can't you're right."
~ Henry Ford, American carmaker

This opening quote always resonated with me since I first heard it from my elementary school softball coach. I admit, at 10 years old, it was a little bit over my head, but something stuck. I remember the day well. After school softball practice where I played for a team called 'The Giants', which I realize in hindsight is oxymoronic as we were anything but gigantic in any stretch of the imagination!

Team sports were something I was always drawn to, but rarely got an opportunity to participate in as I was raised by a single mother with limited resources for such pursuits. This time, however, I could get myself to and from practice and I would mow lawns and do odd chores for extra pocket money to pay the dues. From this initiative you'd think I was pretty awesome at playing the game. Truth was, I wasn't. I had a real problem with making contact with the ball. In other words, I always struck-out. When I did manage to hit the ball, it seemed to land right in the glove of the opponent and I was sent back to the dugout with my tail between my legs.

During one practice though, my coach observed and came over and said, "Do you think you can hit a home run?"

"No," I said in a matter of fact way.

"You're right."

"You'll never be able to hit that ball for a homer or even get to second I imagine, don't you?"

"I guess," I muttered, wondering why he was picking on me.

"It's true, if you don't even consider it's possible, you might as well go warm the bench," as he pointed to the dugout.

As I went to turn and put the bat down and settle in for some bench warming, he quipped "What if you believed you could?"

"What?" I said slightly confused now.

"Uh-huh. If you needed to believe something about yourself, so you knew it was possible, what would it be?" He looked straight at me and I looked around at everyone else, yep, they were all looking at me.

I stood there in what seemed like a moment in time which was forever fixed, as if a stick pin was holding it into place on the corkboard of life for everyone to view as I searched my thoughts for something, anything possible.

Light bulbs sparked, "That it *was* possible, sir."

"Anything is possible if you believe it is."

"Do you believe that?" a wry smile stretched across his unshaven chin.

"Yes. Yes, I do." It was as if I was watching a feel-good, inspiring, made for television, afterschool special, as I began to believe it was possible.

The memory of this is vivid and significant to me and I believe this was the foundation of the 'can-do attitude' I've taken forward in my life. It was only a thought I held about my abilities based on what I had done before which was holding me back from becoming what I wanted to be—a winner.

"To succeed, you must first believe you can." Michael Korda. Novelist.

Beliefs are at the core of our organizing principles that determine our experience of life. These are not the religious beliefs that support our spiritual faith. Core beliefs are the central hub of our intrapersonal wheel from which all life radiates. There is no point in arguing the validity of your belief as being right or wrong, good or bad, true or false. The belief is always true to the believer. You just need to ask yourself, "Does it serve me to believe this thought?"

Medical students learn, albeit in passing, how the mind affects the body. With the two parts of the mind being understood as the conscious and the unconscious mind, you can also begin to understand processes and purposes. The human mind can be viewed as having two main functions: **THINKING** and **PROVING**. What the thinker thinks, the prover proves. For example, you can think about anything at all, however, the prover has no choice. Whatever you think, your mind will arrange information to prove that thought to be true.

Take for example the placebo effect. In the book *Biology of Belief*, scientist Bruce Lipton refers to this as the 'belief effect' which determines how the power of a belief affects our biology. Literally taking it 'out of the mind' and the perception that it is only a phenomenon that happens to only the most suggestible of patients. As he says, "The placebo effect is quickly glossed over in medical schools so that students can get to the real tools of modern medicine like drugs and surgery. This is a giant mistake. The placebo effect should be a major topic of study in medical school and should be used to train doctors to recognize the power of our internal resources."

A good example of this is if a person believes themselves to be stupid. They will sort and filter incoming data they take from their environment in such a way to prove that it is true. They will act and react in a specific way that makes it true. If you believe you will always be poor, life is unfair, weight loss is hard, you are no good, you will find ways of justifying, perceiving, finding evidence for the reality of these beliefs and thereby make it true.

Now if you are thinking "I don't believe it," I am not surprised! Our beliefs extend from the mind and are experienced as egocentric trappings like a maze of thoughts. Take some time to consider this idea and these trappings will start to evaporate and you wake up to the trance phenomenon you have been living.

Huh? I hear you cry. What this means is that your mind is made up of an internal map of reality, where the core principle that organizes stored information is your beliefs. They fundamentally are thoughts, but they run so unconsciously at times, you never think that you can believe something different than you do. This results in a feeling of disbelief or at worse, denial and perhaps even some anger as the veil of your illusion begins to fall away.

Our Internal Map of Reality

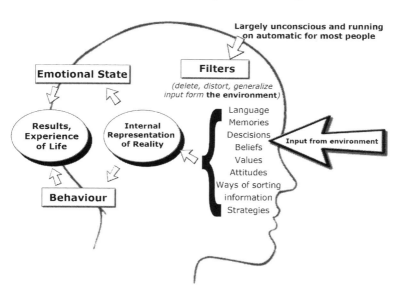

So if you believe you can become a winner, life is a wonderful adventure and people are inherently good and mean well, you will make this true for you. Our external realities are projections or mirrors of our internal realities. This is why everyone has their own subjective perception of reality. How you see the world is unique to you, and the core of your experience of life, is dependent on what you are thinking.

Our thoughts are real things to our mind. Our thoughts affect our feelings which affect our behaviors. This means we are self fulfilling and you can change your experience of life by changing your thoughts. By understanding these functions, filters and processes you can begin to bring them into the cold light of day and change anything that doesn't serve you.

In her book *Emotional Options*, Mandy Evans clearly explains the power of our mindset: "The choices you make and actions you take when you are afraid lead down a different road from the choices and actions you take when you are happy. The solutions you find to a problem when you feel guilty will not be the same ones you come up with when you feel at peace."

How powerful are your beliefs to shape your experience of reality? There is nothing more powerful than a belief believed. Take the Baylor School of Medicine study published in 2002 in the *New England Journal of Medicine* by Dr Bruce Moseley. He wanted to discover which of the surgical procedures he used with patients was most effective so they were divided into three groups to research. Group one had the damaged cartilage in their knee shaved away and group two had their joint flushed to remove material causing inflammation. The third and final group had a fake surgery. In every aspect the third group received pre and post-operative advice and care. During the procedure they had the standard incisions made as if they were having the actual surgery, so in every way it was just as the first two groups received, except it was fake.

In the findings of the study, each group improved equally and measurably. The outcome of the study was clear and Dr Moseley concluded that his skill as a surgeon had no benefit on his patients despite there being over 650,000 surgeries annually for arthritic knees at a cost of over $5,000 each, it was the patients' belief in the procedure and his ability that was effective. The most effective component was belief; the placebo effect.

Some of you may be thinking that what you believe is what you believe and you cannot change what you believe. But what is a belief? It's a thought you think, which you accept 100% at an emotional level as a truth. That is all it ever was. The truth of the matter is you can believe anything you want to believe. Nothing in this world comes with meaning inherently attached to it. You provide the meaning, so you might as well make it good!

For example: you can take two people and stand them side by side. Now take two glasses of ice cold water and splash it in their faces. One person may react badly and scream "YOU JERK!" the other may react as though it was a delightfully refreshing tryst! The ice water has no meaning, except for the meaning given to it by the person.

Some clients would say this means I'm lying to myself. My answer is always, "Well, you are lying to yourself anyway, might as well make it mean something good."

How does this apply to your transformation? By being aware of limiting thoughts, beliefs and meanings you apply / have applied to different things, experiences, circumstances, situations, potentials and possibilities, you are empowered to change them to something that will help you to achieve your goal.

Often people think that transformation takes willpower.

The truth is: *will power is a myth*.

Belief Power vs. Willpower—no contest! Belief power is a thousand times stronger than willpower. Harness the power of belief with all the principles and strategies in this book and it won't be long before you will become the better version of you. The most powerful way to end emotional eating is by increasing your awareness and establishing a belief system that becomes a part of you—the future you, healthy, happy and the perfect weight right for you. This is the authentic expression of you; who you really are, without limitations.

Four core beliefs that fit, healthy people have about food:

Core beliefs 1—Food is building material, the construction material of the body.

Affirmation—*"I will become what I eat as the food I eat becomes the cells, organs and tissues of my body."*

Core belief 2—Food is for fuel.

Affirmation—*"I will be as energetic as the fuel I put in my bodily engine."*

Core belief 3—Food is for nourishment.

Affirmation—*"Nutritious foods contain every thing I need for perfect health."*

Core belief 4—Food is for stoking the metabolic fire.

Affirmation—*"When I feed myself nourishing food when I am hungry, it regulates my metabolism and optimizes fat loss."*

Adopting these types of beliefs could transform your relationship with food. These core beliefs are unemotional beliefs about food that are essentially saying: "It's just food, it's just fuel."

It strips away the intense feelings we associate with food; when you change your beliefs and affirm a new mindset and attitude towards healthy living, food begins to lose its emotional pull over you.

The above core beliefs are helpful, but balance is key to ensure long term happiness and in not depriving yourself of the enjoyment and social rewards that go along with food. Consider some of these beliefs which support long term happiness:

Beliefs for balance, happiness and long term success:

1. I eat with an aim for total satisfaction, because I eat what I prefer.

2. I'm totally conscious and aware of my beliefs about food and the reasons I eat.

3. When I feel stressed or depressed I have alternative ways to manage with those feelings.

4. Healthy food that helps me burn fat and build muscle can be prepared in delicious ways.

5. I realise that food can be one of life's great pleasures and that depriving myself of foods I enjoy is unfulfilling and problematic.

6. I don't have to be perfect, if I listen to my body, hear, understand and respond to its needs I know I will get results.

7. I know that there is no such thing as forbidden, wrong or bad foods—there is just different food with different nutritional qualities.

8. When I take care of myself, I feel great.

9. Everything I eat will have some affect on my body, but I realise that what I eat once in a while doesn't impact me that much.

10. I honour my health, my hunger, my satisfaction and focus on the way things feel to me.

11. What is most important is that I change my relationship with myself and with food. I am aware about what I say to myself, to others, what I think, what I focus my attention on and repeat consistently to myself. I understand and have great respect for the power of habits.

12. My body is the result of the thoughts I think, my feelings about it and how I treat it.

Your beliefs are the conclusions you've decided about your concept of yourself, your abilities and capabilities, your body, other people, the world and your place in the world. Beliefs are programs that run as part of your hardwired mind, running automatically in the background by the unconscious mind. Beliefs act as a roadmap to navigate you through life and help you to make sense of your reality, the events, people and situations you encounter.

Your beliefs are fundamental to shaping your perceptions of reality as they take in stimulus from your environment through your senses such as sight, hearing, smell, touch and taste and make sense of these messages. Our beliefs influence and shape everything about us in our lives, even that which happens beneath our awareness at a cellular level. Amazingly, our beliefs have the power to determine our biology.

The power of the person's belief can affect the way their body reacts. In another scientific study, patients were given morphine over the course of a week but on the final day instead of morphine they were given a saline solution. The patients experienced the same level of pain relief despite not receiving any morphine on the final day whatsoever. The patients' beliefs created the pain relief.

This means that you can influence everything down to the way you heal or metabolize energy by tapping into your inherent ability to do so. If you believe that you can, *you can* optimize this process, changing the shape of your body with your beliefs. For example, if you believe that you have a slow metabolism, you will have. If you believe that your metabolism is functioning optimally—it will.

A belief is more than just thinking positively. It's about accepting what you think as truth 100% at an emotional level. Beliefs change all the time—you can change your beliefs with understanding that *you can change them*. Think about what you believed when you were a child: like Santa Claus or maybe about something you thought you'd never learn how to do, like to ride a bike or to tie your shoes. Look at what you believe now. Beliefs can change in a moment of insight, or by practising techniques which condition the mind into establishing new beliefs and creating a knowing. When you know something, there is no trace of doubt.

Limiting beliefs are a cognitive distortion. They are neither true nor false, they just are thoughts and you can believe them or not. If you believe them and you are aiming for transformation of your relationship with your body and with food, you will need to think again and break down these limiting beliefs so you can choose healthy beliefs that serve and support you.

One of the key ways we are affected by stress is through the limiting beliefs we hold. It has been suggested that 90% of all disease is caused by stress and 100% of all stress is caused by limiting beliefs.

In a potentially stressful situation, people react differently and this is directly linked to what meaning and beliefs they have attached to the situation or stimulus. For example, public speaking—one person may become exhilarated by the prospect of getting up in front of others yet another person would be absolutely terrified by the prospect. It is not the public speaking itself that is the problem, it's the belief about public speaking that is creating the substantial difference.

If a belief you hold causes you to interpret situations in your life in a way that creates a feeling of stress then you are engaging your body's 'fight/flight' response. The prolonged consequence of this will affect the body in a negative way and your health will be compromised. The 'fight/flight' response is a primitive survival instinct that kicks in whenever we are in a dangerous situation—*whether real or imagined*.

We all know that prolonged or chronic stress isn't healthy for us. When we go into the 'fight/flight' response, the stress hormone cortisol is secreted into the bloodstream. This hormone promotes weight gain and some studies have shown that stress and elevated cortisol tend to cause fat deposition in the abdominal area. This fat deposition has been referred to as "toxic fat" since abdominal fat deposition is strongly correlated with the development of cardiovascular disease including heart attacks and strokes.

To facilitate your body to return to its healthy, default, natural weight, the body needs to be in an optimal state where it is functioning normally. This change begins with your beliefs about things in your life which are causing feelings of stress within the body. Remember, stress is not created by something outside of ourselves—it's not the public speaking that is the problem, it is our thoughts and our beliefs about it that makes the problem.

When exploring limiting beliefs look at the areas of your life where you are getting the most negative results. Again, be honest with yourself and look for the things you say to yourself when things have gone wrong or look bleakest. You're not looking for things you should believe about yourself. If that were really true, you would be creating them in your life already.

Beliefs run unconsciously beneath the surface of awareness until you bring them to the surface to examine them. Limiting beliefs such as "I have a slow metabolism", "eating healthily is hard work", "losing weight is hard work", and "I am not good enough", are creating results in your life you do not want. In order to shift these, you need to dismantle them and believe something more resourceful. Remember, the thinker thinks and the prover proves.

Now let's work on creating new resourceful beliefs that support your goal of transforming your relationship with your body and food so you can create a happier, healthier more relaxed version of you.

To do this, get a piece of paper and begin to ask yourself some questions and open up to what you can discover. Write down your limiting beliefs and create a counter-resourceful belief you'd like to have instead. You may want to use the companion workbook available through the website at www. eatguiltrepentrepeat.com

Complete the following sentences:

I am _____

People are _____

The world is _____

My body is _____

Food is _____

Losing weight is _____

Exercise is _____

Eating healthily is _____

Feel free to look at any area of your life where you are not getting the results you want. Remember, your answers are not what you think the answer should be, but what it really is.

A common stumbling block to creating new, resourceful beliefs is wanting to keep the old beliefs even though they result in outcomes you do not want. *Please be very clear that this is not possible.* The definition of insanity is doing the same thing over and over in the same way and expecting to get different results. There's no way to change your results other than to change the contents of your internal map of reality and a key component of that map is what you believe.

Once you know what your core limiting beliefs are and have made the decision that you want different results than you are currently creating, the next step is to decide which beliefs would be more resourceful and whereby would create the results you do want.

Dismantling Limiting Beliefs

You can use the following questions below to dismantle or challenge any limiting belief you hold. By doing so you bring your limiting beliefs into the cold light of day and expose them for what they really are: thoughts you think are true. But these thoughts do not need to be true for you. It's not worth arguing whether a thought is good or bad; remember they are only beliefs that are resourceful or unresourceful or limiting or supporting.

What is the limiting belief?

Is it true?

Can you absolutely know that it is true?

What happens when you believe that thought?

What feelings do you notice?

Where in your body do you feel those feelings?

What pictures, images, movies play in your imagination?

How do you react to other people when you believe that thought?

How do you try to cope with that? (alcohol, food, etc)

When was the first time you remember thinking this thought?

What does believing this thought give you? (safety, protection etc)

What would happen if you didn't believe that thought?

Is there anything you think you cannot do when you believe that thought?

Who would you be without that thought?

What is the opposite of that thought? "I am no good" becomes "I am good"

Is the opposite thought any more or less true than the first one?

How do you know?

What does that mean?

By looking in the opposite direction of what you believe is true, you will find new learning hiding. It can feel tedious to challenge our unconscious core principle beliefs, however, if you lean into it you will begin to discover that by challenging limiting beliefs you give yourself the flexibility to choose what you want to believe instead.

Everything You Think is an Affirmation

What you've learned so far about how beliefs shape your perception of reality is crucial. As you've discovered, everything you think is an affirmation. The definition of what an affirmation is: *Something declared to be true; a statement or judgment* (whether positive or negative). The affirmations that we use reflect the beliefs that we hold and beliefs are the rules we live by, so these rules end up causing us to make ourselves right about that belief. (Thinker, Thinks—*Prover, Proves!)*

What is important to know is that by becoming aware of your thoughts you are empowering yourself to have choice in what you affirm as true in your life. You can create supportive affirmations for yourself which reflect what you want. Like new resourceful beliefs, they are powerful instructions to your mind to help to guide you to what you want.

You can create your own affirmations then put them in your awareness with an external reminder so you remember to think and repeat them often. Negative thoughts that are unsupportive can happen and you'll recognize this with your awareness, and whenever this happens you can use this negative thought like an alarm bell alerting you to repeat your supportive affirmation. Write your affirmations down, type them up, print them and keep them where you can see them.

When writing an affirmation, it's most effective if you write it as if it is already happening, it is accomplished and it's already true. Since it is already accomplished, you know it and feel it in your body at a deep level of understanding. Fake it until you make it! This creates a compelling instruction for your unconscious mind to create it for you and it feels good!

There is power in stating "I am" at the start of all your intentions and affirmations. When you say "I or I am" you are saying this as an identity statement, which serves as a very compelling belief for your unconscious mind to adhere to. What we hold as a truth in our mind, attached to our identity is a powerful statement of certainty that must be rectified as evidence and materialized in your reality. Your mind understands this as factual and already accomplished. It will find ways to make this true in your supporting feelings and deeds. You will also be inclined to see possibilities and potentials with this supporting belief.

By using I am THAT (whatever that may be) I am, you are reaffirming this as a truth.

Below are some resourceful and supportive affirmations / beliefs you could adopt or customize for yourself. When thinking these affirmations imagine you are exhaling your intention for this truth and as you are inhaling you are receiving this truth. Remember, I am is the most powerful of all words as it is who you are. You experience life as you are not as it is.

For example:

Breathe out "I am perfect health."

Breathe in: "I am."

- ✓ I am natural weight that is right for me, I am.
- ✓ I am successful and reaping the rewards of my action, I am.
- ✓ I am perfect health, I am.
- ✓ I am well-being, I am.
- ✓ I am Love, I am.
- ✓ I am Joy, I am.
- ✓ I am perfect peace, I am.
- ✓ I am wealth, I am.
- ✓ I am prosperity, I am.
- ✓ I am abundance, I am.
- ✓ I am fruitful, I am.

- ✓ I am motivation, I am.

- ✓ I am whole, I am.

- ✓ I am energetic, I am.

- ✓ I am authentic, I am.

- ✓ I am commitment, I am.

- ✓ I am courage, I am.

- ✓ I am discipline, I am.

- ✓ I am mastery, I am.

- ✓ I am reverence, I am.

- ✓ I am worthy, I am.

- ✓ I am trust, I am.

- ✓ I am integrity, I am.

- ✓ I am faith, I am.

- ✓ I love and accept myself just as I am.

- ✓ I am worthy of good things and a good life, I am.

- ✓ I am thankful, I am.

- ✓ I am safe, I am.

- ✓ I am beauty, I am.

- ✓ I am contented, I am.

This pattern of affirming is taken from the contemplation meditation yogic mantra Soham or Sohum, which is a reflection of the sound of the breath and means "I am that" (So = "I am" and Hum = "that"). Here, "that" refers to all of creation. In meditation, you breath in on So and exhale on Hum. Using this pattern, you will focus the mind intentionally and your breath will become an anchor.

It's easier than you may think to adopt a new belief. All you need to do is focus on it as often as possible and in every way you can think of. Once you have chosen what you want to believe, based on the results you want to have, you can begin to adopt this new way of thinking about yourself, about others and your life.

By doing this, you will automatically begin to create new results. Remember, your thoughts are real things to the mind—they affect the way you feel and that affects the way you act or react in different situations.

To install a new belief, you have to start feeding it into your mind, over and over, while wiping the old belief out of your mind whenever it pops up. A thought that seems true to you is only a belief that you have let run automatically—you've not brought it out into the cold light of your awareness and examined it for exactly what it is: *A thought you accept as truth*.

The only reason the old belief seems true is that you have focused on it for so long and assumed that it was true. This makes it play out in reality, which of course makes you focus on it more, which makes it play out . . . on and on, in a self-reinforcing cycle.

Focus on this new belief. Think about it while meditating, while driving, while showering, before you go to sleep, before you arise, as often as possible. Doing so may bring up old and uncomfortable feelings and thoughts, so be prepared for that—the old belief will literally fight for its life. Don't let that bother you. Just keep focusing on what you want.

Create a vivid and compelling movie in your mind of yourself getting the result of the new belief, and feeling happy and satisfied by it—the more real and alive the movie, the better the result. Whenever you find yourself thinking about the old, limiting belief, immediately switch your focus to the movie of the new belief. At first this will take effort and may seem awkward, but over time it will become more and more natural and effortless. Eventually, the new belief will be part of you.

Muster as much positive emotion to support your new belief and intention. Feel it as already accomplished. How would it feel to have your desire realized? Would you feel happy, confident, peaceful or contented? Would you have more energy and motivation? Feel it now. Feelings impress the unconscious mind with your desire. The unconscious mind sees you as you believe yourself to be.

Neville Goddard was an influential Metaphysics teacher and New Thought author who said, "To impress upon the unconscious with the desired state you must assume the feeling that would be yours had you already realized your wish. Therefore, when you know what you want, you must deliberately focus your attention on the feeling of your wish fulfilled until that feeling fills the mind and crowds all other ideas out of consciousness."

Challenge all limiting beliefs by using these exercises and dismantle their validity, looking at them from different perspectives. You can also reinforce a new, resourceful belief by reading books by people who share this new belief and way of thinking, socializing with like-minded people, or find a mentor who will help you to establish these new beliefs.

Some limiting beliefs that are beneath your awareness will pop up when you least expect it. It could come up as a judgement you find yourself making against another person, for example: "Look at her; she acts like she knows everything." A judgement you hold against another is a form of a limiting belief that can point you toward a life lesson you can grow from inside of yourself. The world we see and experience comes from inside of us. This means we see the world as we are, not as it is. It's a projection of all the values, generalizations, decisions, judgements and beliefs you've learned along the way. Consider the world and others a mirror. Whenever you have a strong emotional reaction or a negative one based on other people or things outside of yourself, you know it's reflecting back on you a potential lesson or learning that you can grow out of.

Let it be okay that you don't believe it now, that there is a learning curve. Change is a process and changing beliefs can happen at a moment's insight, or by way of repetition and this is done by practising—thinking of the new, resourceful belief, and how this will change everything as if it's already true to you in your imagination. It is already accomplished and just waiting for you. However long this process takes, it is worth undertaking. There is a big difference between being an unconscious automatic response mechanism and living consciously with intention to create the results you want in life.

You are, in fact, already an expert at creating what you believe and focus on. It's just that you did not intentionally choose what you currently believe and focus on. Instead, your beliefs and what you focus on are operating unconsciously and automatically. As long as things continue in this way, you will continue to create the same results you are getting now.

Make a commitment to yourself to be a conscious creator of your reality you desire. Your only limit to what you can achieve is determined by you and the action or lack of action you take.

Action Steps:

1. Identify and dismantle any limiting beliefs you currently hold.

2. Create a list of core beliefs you want to adopt.

3. Create powerful "I am" statements and repeat them first thing in the morning before you get out of bed and last thing at night before you fall asleep.

4. Create a compelling vision or movie of your new belief and play it over and over again.

5. Feel this as already achieved.

6. Make a commitment to be a conscious creator of your life.

Chapter 6—Attraction is Action

"If you do not know where you are going, you'll end up someplace else."
~ Yogi Berra, American major league baseball player and manager

In this process you're beginning to understand how your mind works, how with your awareness, your beliefs, decisions and desire you can achieve your goals. It really is possible for you to have what you want in life. There is a way of thinking and acting that will lead to the outcome you want.

With the popularity of the movie "The Secret" bringing awareness and interest into the Law of Attraction, I want to address some common misconceptions about the power of positive thinking and Law of Attraction. First what is the Law of Attraction? What it means is *like attracts like* or you get what you think about; whether you like it or not—your thoughts determine your results.

There are two ways to approach the Law of Attraction. One is from a 'metaphysical' point of view, the other is from a scientific point of view. It really does not matter which way you look at it, what matters is how you use it to your best advantage to create results.

If you Google "Law of Attraction" over 3-million results are listed. There are sites which will sell you advice on how to order up and "manifest" your desire from the Universe or cosmic menu. A lot of people seem to think that all they have to do is think, dream, wish and pray and everything they want will come to them. There is an array of "how to manifest" or "how to be prosperous" books, seminars and information available out there that tout this formula where you focus on it, pray about it, tell your spirit guides, angels or the Universe about it and it will happen.

This just simply isn't accurate or substantial enough for you to create what you want. I realize we have discussed about how your thoughts are real things because they really affect you—your feelings and your actions are preceded by a thought, whether you are aware of it or not. But it's simply not enough to just wish for things you want, feel as though you already have them and expect your ideal body, your dream partner, that fabulous new job and a dump truck full of money to be delivered to you. The essential missing ingredient is action.

What is essentially happening when you focus your mind on what you want, and you think about it often, is that you create powerful motivation inside, such as good feelings and energy to take action to get what you want. When you focus on what you don't want, what you want to avoid, what you lack, what is missing, what you can't do, all the things you don't like, guess what? You find more of it. Not only will you not feel good when you focus your mind on all the negativity around you—you will create negativity within you and you will act or react in a way that creates more of this. Also, as you've learned, your belief systems are magnets for acting and reacting in certain ways, giving you outcomes that respond in kind to what it is you believe.

By focussing on what you want, what you already have and can be thankful for in your life, the qualities within yourself that you can love and appreciate just as they are, creating compelling, vivid mental imagery and repeating it often, you will feel good, you will have more energy and you will be open to potentials and possibilities you would have otherwise missed. It really is as simple as that.

Take action steps to form a kick ass goal:

STEP 1 Know where you are

STEP 2 Know where you want to be

STEP 3 Take **ACTION**

STEP 4 Evaluate the results of your action

STEP 5 Based on your evaluation, refine your **ACTION**

STEP 6 Keep repeating steps 3, 4, and 5 until you get what you want

You are creating your reality. It is not coming from outside of you. Outer circumstances are a factor in your success, but they are a small factor. The only things you can control are your thoughts, feelings and behaviors. Everything else is outside of your control. The real power comes from inside your head. If there is one stumbling block that absolutely must be removed if you are to become successful in creating transformation or whatever success is for you, it is the idea that your environment determines your results. How you focus your mind and how you act determine your results. Please don't ever forget that.

Principles of success:

- You are responsible for what you create (yes everything!)
- There is a certain way to think and act that will get you any particular outcome you want
- There is always a price to pay to have anything in life
- This isn't magic, what you focus on causes you to know what action to take and motivates you to take it

Basically, your thinking affects your feelings and this will affect your behavior. A good example of this comes from when I wanted a dog. I had not owned a dog as an adult and really wasn't sure what type of dog would fit in with our lifestyle. There were a few things I needed to explore, so I did some research on different breeds to understand their tendencies and their dispositions. I knew a few things I didn't want. This helped me define what I did want. (See what I did there?) It was things like, size; we needed a small to medium-sized dog as our house wasn't that big and we didn't want the dog to take up the room like another piece of furniture. It had to like cats or at least, get used to living with one, because we already had a cat and didn't want a chaser.

As I focussed on what I wanted, I imagined what it would be like to be living together in our house and even went around to several dog shelters to see if we could adopt one. What happened made me realize the power of Law of Attraction in action. Everywhere I went I noticed dogs, dogs, dogs. All types of dogs! Big ones, small ones, yappy ones. Dogs were coming out of the woodwork. Where did all these dogs come from? It wasn't magic. I did not magically manifest all these dogs into existence through the sheer power of my thinking about it. What happened was *I was open to noticing things I would have otherwise filtered out of my awareness.*

Our conscious minds are limited in terms of the number of things we can be aware of at any given moment. Neuroscientists suggest that we are aware of up to ten bits of information taken in through our senses at any given moment. So by filling my mind with thoughts of what I wanted, my mind as the goal seeking mechanism it is, sought out all the opportunities and potentials I would have otherwise missed. This applies to everything in your life, including you changing your relationship with your body and with food so you can return to a healthy, ideal weight.

Jack Canfield is the best-selling author of *Chicken Soup for Soul* books and during one of his seminars he had this great way of illustrating how this all works. A volunteer stands up and plays the role of the goal and Jack tries to get to the goal from the other side of the room. The volunteer's job is to give Jack feedback as he takes action, by saying either "on course" or "off course." When Jack is moving toward the goal, they say "on course," and if he veers away, they say "off course." Just by listening to the feedback and responding, Jack always makes it to the goal.

Sometimes, though, Jack just stands in one place and after awhile asks the volunteer, "Why aren't you saying anything?" The volunteer replies, "Because you haven't moved. I can't give you feedback if you don't move." As obvious as this is, most people don't stop to think that they can't get any feedback about what to do next if they don't take some sort of action.

Sometimes during this exercise Jack is told so many times that he is off course that he breaks down, sobbing. "I can't take it anymore. This is so hard. You're so critical. I give up." Many people, when the feedback they get is something other than "on course," just fall apart and quit. You have to see the feedback you receive as valuable information, no matter what it is. It's all just corrective guidance.

Sometimes when Jack is going off course over and over and the volunteer is having to say "off course, off course," over and over, Jack stops and gets mad. "Nag, nag, nag! Get off my back. Can't you say something positive?" This is the "kill the messenger" syndrome. How many times have you gotten mad at the source of feedback, instead of just learning from it, re-evaluating, and taking a new and hopefully more effective action?

Finally, sometimes Jack stays off course, and continues to get more and more off course, no matter what the volunteer says. In other words, some people just won't listen to feedback. They think they know better, that the feedback is wrong, or that they don't need feedback because they just know inside what to do.

Valuable information might be all around them, but they won't listen. They stubbornly keep on going the wrong way.

Know where you are, know where you want to be, take action, find out what happens, re-evaluate and improve the action, and take action again. Every person who has ever succeeded at anything has done it in this exact way. All the fancy ideas and techniques in the Universe are useless unless you understand and follow these basics. If you've tried to achieve something in your life in the past, and it didn't work, it's because you didn't follow these six steps, and keep following them until you got what you wanted.

In order to set a kick ass goal that will really work, you need to define your main purpose which summarizes your intention, how you know it is possible, and that there is a price to pay for everything in exchange for what you want. Then be as specific as you can and frame the targets as if they are already true for you, and begin with 'I or I am'. Statements framed in the identity context are the most powerful! Now be specific about what you will give in return for this. Then set the date for completion of this goal. Goals without deadlines are just wishes. Also, be flexible in the 'how' this can happen, so add in something like 'or something better' because you may not get specifically what you want (aim high!), so be open for how this will be fulfilled according to your highest potential.

Example: "My main purpose is to feel more positive about myself and change my relationship with food to a healthy one. This is possible because I practice changing my thoughts to focus on what I want and am open to the potential and possibilities that guide me towards the right action to take. This means I have a healthy relationship with myself, my body and with food. I am letting go of past conditioning that no longer serves me. I love and accept myself just as I am. In return for this I will continue to learn, grow and transform myself even if it's a little uncomfortable to do so at times. Reaching all my goals, or something better by [date], knowing that any setback I experience during this time is only feedback and a normal part of changing."

Type up your own and put it someplace you will see it and read it every day. Now, **LET IT GO**. What this means is if you fret, worry, stress, feel the lack and act as it is always out of your reach, you are unconsciously pushing the goal away from you. This is probably the biggest lesson to learn. Have faith that it will happen and if it doesn't happen according to your timeframe, don't sweat it. Remember "or something better" allows things to happen exactly as they should at the perfect time they should. If you have faith in the process and you are moving towards what you want, you will notice opportunities and potentials along the way, pointing you to the next choice point to reveal to you an action step to take. Trust this is part of the process. Keep going. Just keep swimming. Most people want their desire right now. If you are impatient, you only emphasize the lack in your life, which impresses the lack in the mind. The fun is in the process especially when you know how kick ass it's going to be when it is finally realized. Let go and know it will happen at the perfect time. It will when you are ready, open, accepting and allowing the flow of abundance into your life. Expect miracles.

If you become disheartened, frustrated and feel unmotivated, then just leave it for the time being. Be open to discover whatever you need to so you can learn, grow and clear it out so you make room for the new in your life. This is a time for self care and exploration. Sometimes we have to stay still in order to move forward. As cliché as that sounds, it's true. Just get out of your own way and surrender to the process of creation.

Everything you do to move yourself forward to your potential is success. If you've ever heard that success is buried in the garden of failure, or if you've experienced this first hand you will know what I mean. I sure know what it means, I have been there and got the T-shirts! The book you hold in your hand comes from a series of failures. Some of these failures have been so profoundly agonizing, they stripped back the layers of my ego to expose all the fears, shortcomings, limiting beliefs and pain residing beneath the surface that I hadn't come to terms with and was in denial about. I had to let go of these things, before I was able to be the person who writes a successful book. Does that make sense?

Everyone can relate to having things not go the way they would have wanted. Perhaps you had a failed relationship. Perhaps a job you wanted or had didn't work out the way you hoped. It is only in hindsight you can appreciate that what happened to you, although you didn't choose it to go that way, turned out for the best. When we are experiencing it in that moment, it's hard to understand how this too will be okay eventually, maybe not right now, but eventually. When the student is ready, the teacher will present itself and this is a life lesson. You may not have been ready for it before, but when you are, you will. There is nothing more powerful than an idea whose time has come. With that trust and faith, you will reach what you reach for.

If you would have told me 20 years ago, one day I'd be a therapist who helps people overcome their problems and I'd have written a self help book, well, I would have had a good chuckle. Everything that happened to me, once I decided to take intentional action to change my life, pointed me to this exact moment and now I know that I can do whatever I want to do. No longer do I bumble through life unconsciously creating a life that I have to endure. No longer will I settle for less than what I believe I deserve.

Anything I want to be is within my own personal power and reach. I just need to choose it and set into action my intention to create it. So can you.

Take conscious, deliberate action and intend to wake up and begin living the dream. It is said that 'fortune favours those who dare' and it is true. Taking action and living with intention may bring up a lot of junk in your trunk that you need to clear out. Let that be part of your process, knowing that it is only junk and it is within your power to clear it to make room for the new. Do not let the trappings of your egocentric mind keep you thinking that whatever discomfort arises due to you stretching yourself is real. It is only an illusion and this too shall pass, especially when you know it will, sooner with every new goal you stretch yourself to become and as you expand your comfort zone to infinite. Just think of the possibilities!

There is only nothing and in this nothingness is the formless and shapeless, until you think it into existence. Everything comes from nothing and it seemed impossible until someone, just like you, made it possible. You are everything and everything is you. Within you is the power to create anything because everything you create is you. You are only limited by you thinking you are limited. Take off the veil. Turn on your light. Shine.

Action Steps:

1. Create your action plan and begin taking steps towards what you want.

2. Keep repeating the steps until you achieve your goal.

3. Let go of the intention and trust what you want will come if you keep taking action.

Chapter 7—Lean Into Your Transformation

"It's the end of the world as we know it and I feel fine."
~ Lyrics by R.E.M.

Change is a process and can bring up distressing emotions such as fear and resistance. When change is really profound, it will feel as though your whole world is coming to an end. 'It's the End of the World as We Know It', a song by R.E.M. pops to mind here and that's because IT IS!

This is the dying of an old belief system and understanding of yourself as you understood it before. It may be difficult to understand but your fear and your resistance is a good thing. It's an indication that change is coming. Pay attention and keep moving through it. In other words, let it be okay you are feeling uncomfortable.

Nobel Prize winning scientist Ilya Prigogine outlines this natural process of change in complex systems. Humans are a complex system. This process is the principle of chaos and reorganization. This means as a biological system, you are always in a process of irreversible structural changes. What this means for you is that you go into temporary chaos in response to too much input, or your threshold being too low to deal with the stimulus affecting you and it falls apart and reorganizes or reforms at a higher level of functioning.

Consider this: you have a map of your reality—this map includes all the ideas, meanings, experiences, judgements, generalizations, emotions, understandings, learnings, knowledge, beliefs, attitudes and values. This map is our concept of ourselves in relation with everything outside of ourselves in the Universe.

When we experience dysfunctional feelings and behaviors, get stressed out to the point we are causing emotional and mental suffering to ourselves, we are in fact using coping mechanisms to resist our internal map of reality falling apart. We feel ourselves going into internal chaos and we fear that WE are falling apart. We defend to hold onto our current internal map, failing to realize that a new and better map will take its place.

We believe that the map is who we are, rather than just a handy conceptual tool we use to help us through life. We get so used to using our concept of reality when making decisions about what to do, how to feel, how to act, and so on, that we forget it's just a tool and that who we really are is much more. In fact, it's like having an actual map from the turn of the century and trying to figure out a way to go from New York to California, and getting stressed because the map doesn't include information about interstates and highways. It's not we who are deficient, it's our map. Our map isn't who we are. Treating your map as though it is real is like going to a restaurant and trying to eat the menu.

How does this work for you in real life? Firstly you have to accept that chaos precedes change. Whenever you experience chaos or stress in your life, it means your map is unable to handle current stimulus you are experiencing. At which point, you can remind yourself that A) a new map would be pretty handy right now and would in fact solve the problem and B) chaos is a sign that I am getting ready to create a new map and if I get out of my own way its creation will happen easier and faster.

This is a simple process to make inevitable change happen efficiently and without suffering. By clinging to and resisting change you create suffering in your life. Change becomes a pain in the ass and you fear it and you suffer through it. People rarely take responsibility for the chaos or stress they feel in their lives. They project it onto others with blame, "I'm stressed because of my kids/parents/ partner/finances/health/whatever." Blame is the greatest pastime for those who dislike responsibility!

Many people instantly self-medicate whenever they begin to feel stressed. They reach for food, drink, drugs, anything to mask and distract them from what they are feeling. They do not realize that the chaos they feel is a growth opportunity and that by not taking advantage of it they are condemning themselves to repeat the stress and chaos over and over.

Change is a natural process. Here are the steps you can follow to 'let it be okay':

Step 1. Notice and acknowledge that you are in chaos or stress.

Step 2. Realize it is coming from YOU. Stress is not because of something outside of you. Yes there is stimulus or a trigger but it is not the CAUSE.

Step 3. Remind yourself that this is a GOOD thing which means you are in a place of growth to a higher level of understanding.

Step 4. Give acceptance and thanks for this process. Let it be okay that this is happening.

Step 5. Notice how this is happening; if you have resistance, fear or worry, then go back to Step 1.

Consider this in your contingency when preparing for your journey towards transformation. This process is much easier when you build in understandings that at times, it may be difficult and uncomfortable, but if you lean into it and get out of your own way, you'll get there eventually and it will be worth it!

Most self help books never address quitting. They tell you about all the steps you can take to transform your life, but they don't address when people give up. I know from my personal experience that there is no quitting. You never really stop doing anything. What you learn doesn't stop working, you just go back to old ways of thinking and feeling. When you fall back into old patterns, remember that this can be part of the process.

Learning to trust life to teach you what you need is probably one of the hardest lessons there is. It hazards you to give up control of your life and have faith in something bigger to shape your experience of life. I know for me, this was very hard to do.

Consider that in your life you've had many experiences, some good, some not so good. We've already explored how you apply the meaning to everything so you can make it mean whatever it needs to mean for you to feel however you wish to feel. The point is, that when you feel like giving up you can fall back into old familiar patterns of behavior where those old coping strategies you used before, make you feel worse. It is time you recognize that by repeating old patterns you are still needing the lesson they are trying to teach you.

Learn the lesson and move on. There is no quitting you just keep repeating old patterns. To move beyond those old patterns, you need to grow. Challenges are opportunities for growth. Sometimes, we need to be reminded how little time we have to do so. When we find ourselves unable to move forward, let it be okay that is where you are. This is only temporary. Imagine there are lessons from this you may not be able to be aware of at your current level of consciousness. Imagine you can stretch yourself to absorb those lessons, whatever they may be.

By doing so you are actively participating and intending to move forward from your past. Wherever you are right now is where you need to be and you will look back on this time with a greater appreciation for your current mindset.

At this point you can imagine yourself at a crossroad. At this crossroad you have two choices. You can continue to walk down the path that you currently are, repeating the same thoughts, feelings and behaviors which have led you to this point. Doing the same thing in the same way and getting the same results or you can choose another way.

If you stay on the current path then imagine you can shift your gaze as far as you can see down that path. Take steps down this path and notice how it seems to you. Notice how it currently feels to be you with the limitations of your problem. Stretch out all the way to the end of this road to the end of your life where you come face to face with yourself on your deathbed. Get a sense for how this future you represents themselves. How does it look, feel, seem and what are they doing? This is you, where the limiting thoughts, feelings and behaviours are taking you.

If you were to ask the deathbed you to pass on some wisdom, what would they share with you? What do they urge you to know? Take a few moments and allow yourself to fully understand everything that is most beneficial for you to take stock, that we only have a limited number of moments in our life. We never know when those moments will end. This is your future representation by negative age progression. This representation can be useful to hold in your mind whenever you feel like repeating the same old patterns that you know are hurting you.

If this seems morbid or strange considering how our thoughts affect feelings and how the mind doesn't know the difference between what is real and what is imagined, then consider this. You may remember when you were younger a moment where you realized that people die. You may even have experienced the death of a loved one. In a flash you may have felt stricken with an overwhelming urgency of emotion.

We have a tendency to think we have an unlimited amount of time and there's no consequence to our meandering through life. The truth is you have the time you have. When needed, you can remind yourself of the consequence of regret by acknowledging your imagined deathbed personification and their pleas for your action.

People rarely regret taking action, even if it results in failure. I really don't believe in the notion of failure, it's all just feedback. Even if the results are not what you hoped for, it is only the belief that you are a failure that makes you give up. What I do believe is that you regret not having done something. If you do nothing, you will feel as though you've wasted the valuable moments in your life holding onto old patterns that immobilize you.

As you experience the change by doing the work this book teaches you, you will notice how the future you changes. Your life is waiting so don't waste another moment considering anything but that.

Taking in this momentous occasion to take a step towards where you want to go and making a promise to the future you to be aware and responsible for the choices you make from now, which will either lead you to the future you where health and happiness you deserve await you—or lead you away from this you. The choice is yours.

Action Steps:

1. Recognize that change can be uncomfortable, and that it is a good thing.

2. Lean into your transformation with courage.

3. Get out of your own way and allow old systems to fall away.

4. If you are repeating old patterns, then use the negative age progression to feel urgency.

Chapter 8—Live in the Now

"You can destroy your now by worrying about tomorrow."
~ Janis Joplin, American singer

Whether the key to your problem is your relationship with food, yourself or limiting beliefs, there is an element of learning about how to be more present-minded and how you can learn to let go of your negative past that continues to affect and define your present moment and your future.

It may seem contradictory to previous messages that you need to focus your mind on what you want in order to get what you want. The point is, you will think thoughts, that is what the mind does—think thoughts. You can never stop thinking about things. In fact, thinking of nothing is still the thought of something. It's a paradoxical mindset to attempt to be a blank slate. Being mindful means you are no longer victim of the trappings of the mind. Thoughts come and go, but they do not define you. In the space created between stimulus and response is a choice point. This choice point gives you flexibility. So by understanding how to be mindful and when the mind does wander—whether to review the past or plan the future, you do so as a detached observer to this process the best that you can.

What this means, is that you can analyze, review, plan, fantasize, daydream—but be detached from the outcomes. You are *watching with curiosity* the processes of the mind wandering without being directly affected by what you are thinking.

So the principle of thoughts affecting feelings and behaviors is still true, but you have another level of control over this: to allow emotional charges around these thoughts or not. Emotional charges are how thinking those thoughts make you feel—if you think about things going the way you do not want them to in the future, the emotional charge may be stress, worry, concern or fear. If you are thinking something that is supportive, that is positive and supports you in what you want to create in this world then it could mean excitement or anticipation and that's excellent. Either way, you can choose to experience it as the observer, with curiosity, but be detached from outcomes. You can just as well explore potential negative results and consequences from a detached point of view.

All my client's problems exist in either the past or the future. Their problems do not exist in the now. No problems exist in the now. This is because we very rarely experience the now moment as a thought. It is only in hindsight, in review, looking back on something or in the planning or imaging of something that we actually experience a problem.

We either cannot be happy now that things happened the way they did in the past and we want them to be different from how they are, or we want things to be like they were before but they are not. It may be that we expect the future to be like it was before and that's a problem too.

Without even knowing it, we fluctuate between focussing on the past or the future—rarely engaged in our present moment. Since our thoughts are real things, we frivolously waste our precious now moments with this futile exercise of mental gymnastics that changes nothing at all and only reinforces the neurology of the problem!

Cultivating mindfulness will not only help you to bring awareness into your current moment so you are more empowered to make positive choices, it will also help you begin to understand that you are the creator of your experience of life. Everything begins with a thought. The ancestor of every action is a thought— whether you are aware of it or not. Being mindful gives you this awareness so you can take conscious and intentional action.

This puts you firmly in the driver's seat of your life. Here at the start of your journey, knowing exactly where you are, loving and accepting yourself exactly how you are right now, marking yourself on the map of your life in this present moment, you are now ready to head towards where you want to go. With the intention to let go of limiting beliefs and conditioning you have the tools and strategies to do so. Armed with conscious awareness which gives you the power to notice the insights, signs and possibilities along the way to get you to where you want to go.

Let it be okay if you don't know how to do this yet. As you practice and apply these principles into your life this information will become experiential. Learning is a process. Like anything you learn for the first time, it takes practice. Practice makes perfect and permanent.

Mindfulness is something you practice, until it is something you are. The biggest challenge is making the choice to choose to switch off from auto-pilot and be in the now. It is only a choice, but the world is full of distractions—so many things to think of, to plan, to review, to watch on television, to check your phone, to look at your social network feeds, search on the Internet for . . . All of that is so automatic, you probably aren't even aware how compulsive and natural it has become for you to do so. Even more shocking is how unnatural it feels to do nothing at all like just being still, to watch everything with curiosity and be free from judgement.

The Present Moment Is the Only Moment That Never Ends

The benefits of mindfulness practice include improved health, reduction of physical pain and suffering, management of emotional pain such as anxiety, panic, anger, jealousy, grief and shame.

Brenda J. Bentley

Research shows that people who regularly practice mindfulness have a greater appreciation for life, experience activities more intensely where even mundane, repetitive tasks, like washing dishes or driving to work, can take on an extraordinary vibrancy.

One study by Dr Richard Davidson shows that immune system functioning is improved in regular mindfulness practitioners. Over an eight week period, practitioners studied showed an increased response of antibodies to flu vaccination. They also showed an increase of blood flow to the left frontal cortex of the brain which is associated with increased optimism and sense of well-being.

Adopting a daily practice to be still will help you to detach from the mental clatter that your thoughts can create and give you space to choose more empowering thoughts. To help you develop this practice you can download a free audio recording of a short mindfulness meditation from the website www. eatguiltrepentrepeat.com that can help you with cultivating present moment awareness.

This short exercise helps you to take a few moments out of your day to learn how to be more mindful. It may seem simple to just be still and aware, but it is something we rarely are. Cultivating mindfulness and awareness will help you to be more empowered to choose your thoughts more carefully and be less affected by running on autopilot.

You can also use the S.T.O.P. exercise as detailed in an earlier chapter.

S—Stop whatever you are doing

T—Take a few deep breaths and notice the breath as it is, not trying to control the breath just using your breath as an anchor for this present moment

O—Observe your experience—what's happening in this moment in your mind, body and surroundings

P—Proceed by asking yourself, "What is most important to pay attention to right now?"

This strategy can be used with all the other strategies to help you cultivate awareness and be mindful of your thoughts, feelings and behaviors. The purpose of this strategy is to connect with the present moment fully to give you space of empowerment of choice and in this space between stimulus and response, connect with the inner wisdom within you.

Learn to witness and name—this is where you can stand back from your thoughts and watch them with curiosity. You can then 'name' what you notice, whatever you notice—give it a name.

1. Make yourself comfortable

2. Whatever you notice, give it a name. For example, you may first notice your eyes feel tired. Say in your mind, "I notice my eyes are tired." Then wait to see what you notice next. It may be the sound of a passing car, "I notice a car sound."

Using the phrase I notice you will focus your consciousness. Remember consciousness is energy and you need to improve the quality of your consciousness in order to be clear.

Action Steps:

1. Cultivate mindful awareness with a daily practice.

2. Use exercises such as S.T.O.P. and Witness and Name.

Chapter 9—You Are Not Your Past

"The past is behind, learn from it. The future is ahead, prepare for it. The present is here, live it."
~ Thomas S. Monson, American religious leader and author

Part of this process of change means you will need to consider that how you think about the past and its continued affect on you, means you need to let it go completely and for good. This may make some of you shudder to think: "What do you mean let it go? Let it go where? I can't let it go! My past is a part of me! It has made me who I am!" This is where I dare you to consider who you would be without your stories.

The stories we tell ourselves and others become the script for our life. These are all a part of how the mind shapes our realities. The experiences and events of our life, the meanings we attach to them become our reality. We run on autopilot letting our past define our now moments and this is projected out in the future as an expectation. Sometimes this happens beneath the surface of our awareness. We are only aware of the negative results we keep creating or the symptoms of this; like lack of confidence, self worth issues, fear, stress, anxiety, etc.

Just as learning to be mindful and have present moment awareness allows you to detach from the mental clatter our thoughts create, learning to release the negative past and the stories that do not serve you will liberate you to be more clear and present to do so.

By detaching the emotional negative past, you can reprocess any significant emotional experiences in a way that gives you the power to liberate yourself—so that you are no longer experiencing that internal struggle or battling against the intention or purpose of the behavior.

All behavior has a purpose. The problem behaviors you experience have an intention. Our unconscious mind has the sole directive to keep you safe and protected. Regardless of what limiting behaviors you experience in the process, ultimately, this is the underlying driver of limiting behaviors—e.g. lack of confidence or anxiety serves the purpose of limiting you from experiencing anything that would make you feel unsafe or unprotected.

For example, you experience a lack of confidence at the idea of speaking up at the board meeting. You begin to get a feeling of dread inside building up to a feeling of terror. You know you are going to be called on and you imagine how horrible the experience will be with everyone looking at you and judging you. You're going to mess it up—you just know it! You are immobilized by this fear. You decide to make an excuse as to why you cannot attend the meeting and live to fight another day.

This lack of confidence has an intention to keep you from experiencing things that are deemed unsafe or uncomfortable by your unconscious mind. Being human, our primitive reactive processes are about moving us away from pain and towards pleasure. Part of what our unconscious mind does for us is to do this automatically. This is the automatic response mechanism noted on earlier pages.

Memories hold emotion. Or you can say that it is an emotional charge around a memory. What this means is that you can think about something that happened that was upsetting and if you got involved in that memory you could become upset now. If you've ever seen how brain activity is measured, it's like an electrical light show of activity as neurons fire off, you'll understand the term 'emotional charge.'

This is not exclusive to thoughts about the past. You can also do this with the future—if you were to think about something happening in the way you do not want it to happen, you could cause yourself to get worried, concerned or stressed. Thoughts are real things to the mind, it does not distinguish between real or imagined, past or future thoughts, thoughts are real things because they really affect us.

Emotional charges around memories are how the mind stores information that has an instinctual purpose of moving away from pain and towards pleasure—keeping us safe and protected. I refer to these emotional charges as 'adaptive learnings'. Now, not all memories hold emotion and not all memories that hold emotion are adaptive learnings. There are two reasons that a memory would have an emotional charge around it. One reason is that it is an upsetting event such as bereavement. The other reason is that it is an adaptive learning, or as a psychologist would refer to this, a defence mechanism or coping strategy.

Laura came to see me to help her lose weight. She had been overweight for the last 15 years. When we explored her history, it was apparent that her weight gain directly coincided with her marriage. When I asked her if she realized that she had gained weight when she got married and had settled down she acknowledged that she did.

She told me that her husband and his family didn't approve of her. She was constantly putting her needs aside and doing things to try to win their approval, but nothing seemed to work. She was unhappy and indecisive. She felt like she was caught in a fog every time she tried to make a simple decision and didn't trust herself at all to make the right one. She said it was like walking on egg shells all the time, even with herself.

We explored her relationship and she confessed she didn't want to get married. She was an independent person who had a thriving lifestyle in London. Her parents were urging her to settle down and arranged for her to meet a man who they approved of for her to marry. As she came from a traditional Asian culture, this was not uncommon. She explained that although the meeting of her husband was arranged, she was given the choice to say no. She didn't want to say yes and did so reluctantly. She wasn't forced to say yes, but she felt she couldn't say no. Laura wasn't ready for marriage and was resentful for giving up her life to make her parents happy.

As she told me her story, she explained she was very close to her father. When she had left home and finished university, he wanted her to find a husband, but supported her. A few years passed and her father became distant from her. He froze her out emotionally and it was very hard on her. As she remembered how this felt, she was tearful as she explained how important her father's approval was to her. "It hurt really bad when he did that," she wept. She resented marrying to win the approval of her father.

Now she resented her husband for withholding approval. She felt like everything was wrong and she turned to food to escape her feelings. She described her life as living in a cocoon of her husband's world and she felt detached, isolated and lonely. She was numb and said she couldn't figure out what to do to stop her binging.

Laura continued to tell her story and when she was finished I asked her if she had realized before telling me her story that she had so much emotion attached to that memory of her father's rejection. She hadn't realized it was so strong. We worked together to reprocess that emotional charge around that memory so she could release it. From that point we were able to get her to gain some perspective on her father's behavior. She recognized that her father only wanted what was best for her.

He wanted her to be happy and that it didn't make him happy for her to be unhappy. This was the first time she was able to understand how important her happiness was! She also made an astonishing breakthrough when she had an 'ah-ha moment' when she said she had been expecting her husband to fill the void she felt inside from the perceived rejection of her father! From that moment, Laura felt lighter and more at ease and her binge eating behavior stopped.

Laura had unresolved emotional pain that needed to be released. Her binge eating behavior was directly linked to her resentment toward her father and husband. By releasing this emotion, she freed herself from the cocoon she was living in.

You can reprocess information automatically stored by the mind as an adaptive learning so that you do not have automatic responses or internal struggles and can make changes in your life. The aim is to change the way the mind has stored the information. As you can appreciate, we cannot change the past. What we are dealing with is the thought of the past—not the past itself. We can change the meaning and make the emotional charge around a memory neutral or flat so it no longer triggers off the adaptive learnings.

Your struggle with transformation is linked in with either your poor relationship with yourself or with food, maybe a bit of both. It is also about what you believe about yourself, your place in the world and other people in it. Understanding that it is within your personal power to change your life script to something where you can get the results you really want by ending the inner struggle.

It's worth underlining again how important it is that you understand how powerful your imagination is, and how you can use it to make a positive change in your life. This is about using your imagination in a powerful and positive way. You can learn to use your imagination to reprocess the imaginary past. I realize this is probably a way you are not used to thinking. Consider what this means and allow yourself to let it be okay that it all seems unfamiliar. Perhaps you are uncertain. Allow yourself to dare to believe that what you are learning is truer than what you currently believe now.

If you find yourself getting confused just trust your unconscious mind to do it for you—and it will. You just need to turn this entire process over in faith to the part of you that is responsible for it. Be open to allow yourself to let go of limitations in how you can change. If you find yourself being resistant to it, then you know that there is good work to be done!

What is Your Story?

"I am a lover of what is, not because I am a spiritual person, but because it hurts when I argue with reality."
~ Bryon Katie

In order to make something into a 'problem' you have to do one of two things:

1. Compare it to how things used to be and decide they should be that way again, even though they're not.

2. Compare it to how you would like to be and decide it should be that way now, even though it isn't.

In other words, in order to turn a fact of life into a problem to be solved, you first have to create a story about how things should be instead. Our story is the meaning we give to the facts of our life—our interpretation on reality. If we make the facts of our life mean good things about us and the future, we will feel happy about them; if we make them mean bad things, we will feel unhappy about them. Either way, we're the ones ascribing the meaning.

Most of us go through life letting it 'happen to us'. Never considering that the meaning we attach to circumstance is subjective. This means it is our interpretation of what happened that is reality—not the circumstance itself. Remember the example of the ice water? It is the same circumstance, but two different meanings!

Let's play a game, it's called *'what else could this mean?'* Here's how you play. Take any circumstance and attach a meaning to it. For example, if we take the situation where someone gets fired from their job, most may assume that this is a bad thing and they will respond accordingly with a blend of sympathy and encouragement.

But what else could it mean? Here are some plausible options:

- ✓ This is a chance for them to pursue their life's passion.

- ✓ This is an opportunity to develop their skill base and find the right job for them.

- ✓ They will learn and grow from this so they are more wise and experienced.

- ✓ This is an opportunity for a fresh start.

If you practice playing this game, you'll realize that it is possible to apply hundreds of different meanings. After becoming a master of that game, something even more empowering emerges: *what do you want it to mean?*

With this realization you can literally make up the meaning of even the most significant 'facts' of your life. You can begin to deliberately choose the meanings that feel good and empower yourself to take positive action. As I say to my clients: "If you're going to make stuff up, make up good stuff." The way to consistently 'make up good stuff' is to understand and master what cognitive therapists call your 'explanatory style'.

Dr Martin Seligman, psychologist and creator of the Positive Psychology Approach studied optimism. The study shows that people who explained their problems as permanent, personal and pervasive had a completely different experience of life from those who explained their problems as being temporary and specific and didn't take them personally. The benefits of an optimistic outlook are many: optimists tend to be higher achievers and are healthier overall. Pessimism, on the other hand, is much more common. Pessimists tend to give up in the face of adversity or suffer from depression. In his book, *Learned Optimism*, Seligman invites pessimists to learn to be optimists by thinking about their reactions to adversity in a new way by learning a new explanatory style. This explanatory style changes outlook of problems as not personal, not permanent and not pervasive. Problems are explained as not being your fault, temporary and a one-off occurrence. According to Seligman the explanatory style is defined as below:

Personalization: Optimists blame bad events on causes outside of themselves, whereas pessimists blame themselves for events that occur. Optimists are therefore generally more confident. Optimists also quickly internalize positive events while pessimists externalize them.

Permanence: Optimistic people believe bad events to be more temporary than permanent and bounce back quickly from failure, whereas others may take longer periods to recover or may never recover. They also believe good things happen for reasons that are permanent, rather than seeing the transient nature of positive events. Optimists point to specific temporary causes for negative events; pessimists point to permanent causes.

Pervasiveness: Optimistic people compartmentalize helplessness, whereas pessimistic people assume that failure in one area of life means failure in life as a whole. Optimistic people also allow good events to brighten every area of their lives rather than just the particular area in which the event occurred.

Which one are you? Are you an optimist or a pessimist? If you are pessimistic, or even if you think you're an optimist, then try this experiment and change your explanatory style:

1. Think of a problem. Ask yourself: "Why did it go badly?"

2. Explain why it went badly, but this time take out any reference to it being your fault in any way. (This is the first 'p': personalisation.)

3. Now explain what happened again, but as if it were a one-off occurrence with a beginning, middle and end. (This is the second 'p': permanence.)

4. Finally, explain the situation as if it were an isolated occurrence in the otherwise happy, contented experience of your life. (This is the third 'p': pervasiveness.)

5. Notice which of the three changes (personalisation, permanence, pervasiveness) made the biggest impact on your state and begin to rewrite the stories of your life from this new and different point of view.

Learn that you can be the author and editor-in-chief of your story. We all have a story we tell ourselves and others. Did you know that all emotions become memories of emotions after about a half an hour or so? Memories are adjustable. Have you ever played 'Chinese whispers'—where you whisper something to one person and ask them to pass it along—by the time it gets to the end of the line of people, the story has changed. This next exercise is a powerful, life changing exercise—which puts you firmly in the position of author and editor of your life. The following exercise is adapted from the works and teachings of author and counsellor, Rubin Battino.

1. Tell your life story. The way it happened. Write it down. You'll have to do some summarizing as not to write a novel! Tell the story as if you were telling someone you trusted. Then after doing this read it—then write a sentence, phrase or word that is a 'key' or 'moral' to the story.

2. Tell a new story. Tell a new life story where you could go back and write it and live it all over again. There's no boundaries—you are the writer / editor! Then write a sentence, phrase or word that is a 'key' or 'moral' to the story.

3. Now write down how your new life story has changed your future. You may find that the first story is much longer than the second, which is longer than the third. What has changed? What is similar? What have you decided to keep? What was deleted? Did it make any difference to your future?

This exercise is purely a reflective one to help you to realise that you are the only one that can apply meaning over your experience. You can also realize that some experience initially given a negative meaning can be given another meaning that is transformational, pivotal and necessary for growth.

Action Steps:

1. Imagine any experiences that are upsetting to you. Connect with the emotion and imagine releasing it.

2. Ask yourself: What else could this mean?

3. Use the 3-P's when considering what upsetting events mean to you.

4. Become the editor and write and rewrite your story. What is the moral?

5. Consider all your experiences necessary for growth.

Chapter 10—Forgiveness is Freedom

"You know you have forgiven someone when he or she has harmless passage through your mind."
~ Rev. Karyl Huntley

What does forgiving have to do with healing your relationship with yourself and with food? When moving forward from your past stories, you may need to consider forgiveness as a necessary part of the process. Forgiveness gives you the freedom to create a new future without the past's influence. Exploring your life's story, the meaning and concept of yourself, your experiences, the people in it and the part they have played has given you insight as to whether forgiveness is an essential part of your transformation. Forgiveness is the most powerful thing you can do for yourself. It is not something you do FOR someone else. Simply identify the situation to be forgiven and ask yourself: "Am I willing to waste my energy further on this matter?" If the answer is no, then you know you're ready to begin the process of forgiving.

Forgiveness is an act of the imagination that dares you to see things differently. Forgiveness means you give up your destructive and negative thoughts about the situation and believe in the possibility of healing. It dares you to consider that your pain is not the final word on the matter and that you can grow from it. The bottom line is suffering is not good for the soul, unless it teaches you to stop suffering.

Forgiveness is a choice that comes from you. You do not have to forgive but there are consequences for choosing not to. Refusing to forgive by holding on to anger, regrets, resentment and a sense of betrayal can make your own life miserable, create unease and disease in you. When you re-sent, you remember, you re-feel and re-live the pain over and over again in your imagination. Sometimes the grievances and hurt have been so painful you may have thought, "There's no way I can forgive them." These resentments and hostilities can run so deep that forgiveness becomes very difficult. We feel we have a right to our indignation.

What purpose does this serve you? To continue to feel hurt, resentful, angry, bitter, victimized or betrayed? You continue to suffer for what purpose? Forgiveness is not about approval or saying "I'm now fine with what you did to me." It's not about forgetting what happened either. What forgiveness allows you to do is be free from the negative emotional connection to the past.

By referring to previous struggles and using them as reasons for not getting on with your life today, you're assigning responsibility to the past for why you can't be successful or happy in the present. If you choose to withhold forgiveness from yourself, it means you continue to remain the victim held prisoner to your memories of the past.

By choosing to be the victim, you suffer in the illusion that you are the wounded innocent and take a superior position to comfort yourself with being right. You may even gain sympathy from others allowing you to bask in the righteousness of being wronged. Sympathy can act as a salve to the wound, but it's certainly not the cure. Relying on sympathy is like taking pain medication for an infection when what you need is the antibiotic.

We all have our own path to follow. All of us are doing exactly what we know how to do in that moment given the conditions of our lives. This allows you to transcend blaming others. The only antidote to anger and disappointment is to allow yourself to eliminate the expectation that others should treat you like you would treat them. When you judge others, you are not defining them, you are defining yourself as someone who needs to judge. Also, remember how other people mirror the beliefs you hold.

If you choose to forgive, it is not important to tell that person you have forgiven them. Forgiveness has little or nothing to do with the other person because forgiveness is an internal matter. When you forgive you do it for you, not for someone else. That is only and always your choice. The choice to forgive is only and always yours.

To heal yourself and move forward in a life where you are at peace within yourself, you will need to let go of the expectation that you need to be asked for forgiveness. You must accept that this may never happen. People have a way of justifying things because taking responsibility for a wrongdoing can be painful truth. It's easier to blame others and justify their behavior outside of themselves. Remember, blame is the favourite pastime of those who dislike responsibility.

However, living from resentment takes so much effort and energy. It creates a tremendous void in and around us. All the toxic feelings of hatred and resentment stay bottled up inside and eventually seep into all the areas of our life with the result that we become bitter, angry, unhappy and frustrated. Every moment you spend upset, angry or in despair is a moment you've given up control of your life.

Everyone, including you, needs forgiveness. The two most futile emotions in this life are guilt for what has already happened and worry for what might happen. When we think about forgiveness, we think about the wrongdoings that others have done, but what about the wrongdoings you have done to others or to yourself? No one is perfect and we all make mistakes, even unintentionally. It's worthwhile to think of all the times you've hurt, upset, disappointed, lied or betrayed others. Take an inventory and give the gift of forgiveness to yourself.

Everybody has the potential to do hurtful, self destructive and foolish things. You can hurt your loved ones and yourself. You may be hurting right now because of something that you did in the past. Forgiving yourself is in many ways more difficult than forgiving others. When you are unwilling to forgive yourself, you turn the force of your bitterness and anger inward which leads to self-loathing.

If you are withholding forgiveness from yourself, it is impossible to forgive others. Your pain hardens your heart making you hard to love. Forgiveness releases others and yourself from your judgements and criticism. It is not surrender, submission or resignation, but a conscious decision to cease harbouring resentment, regret, guilt and anger any longer. It cleanses your system of the poison that festers and causes suffering.

"Unforgiveness is the poison you drink everyday hoping that the other person will die."
~ Debbie Ford

The above quotation deeply resonated with me through some unpleasant situations I experienced in my life. About five years ago, I decided to start up roller derby in my region of England. I loved roller skating and had participated in competitive speed skating as a child. I noticed there was a resurgence of the sport in the USA where groups of women were forming their own DIY teams. So, I set out to do so here in England. I was involved in the first established club, but it was too far to travel. With a lot of enthusiasm and my skating skills, I set out to establish a club locally. I spent countless hours, labouring in love to train and develop the fledgling sport and the participants. It ended up being a definitive lifestyle for many of the participants. There were growing pains and personal politics that you expect in establishing a new venture trying to garner the cooperation of others in the process. They don't call it 'derby drama' for nothing!

Unfortunately, I became a scapegoat for many of the shortcomings, dramas and difficulties experienced that followed me throughout my derby career. There were a lot of haters hating and some of it was politically motivated to tarnish my reputation. To summarize this, it was the accumulation of negativity fuelled by inexperience in managing others, drama queens, crooked politicians and interpersonal cliques. Due to this, I was unceremoniously dismissed and subsequently rejected by people I thought were my friends.

Overnight, I went from someone who was active in a huge sporting community, with lots of friends and social engagements, to having nothing to do with it. It was one of the most hurtful experiences of my life. When you put so much of yourself into something, you become emotionally invested. I was very attached to this endeavour to the point it became 'who I was' not 'what I did'. It was my world. It was my identity. Buddha says, "The origin of suffering is attachment" and I concur.

The sense of betrayal, the perceived backstabbing, the humiliation of the experience happened in a very public way as my dismissal was announced through social media channels as people carelessly tossed their opinions around. I was angry and resentful. I suffered so much and it was difficult to reconcile the pain in my heart, mind and spirit. There were the people I blamed, as they blamed me. There was the situation connived through gossip vultures and Chinese whispers. I worked hard on letting it all go. To heal the wounds like a dog kicked to the curb, beaten and devastated as the home they once shared rejected them. When the community I had brought together and spent so much time in building with an aim to involve, accept and give those who felt they didn't fit in a place to belong goes and spits you out, well, it's a troubling thing. It felt like high school all over again. I was a social pariah and I felt victimized by all the mean girl politics.

I fell into a depression. The experience seemed to bring up so much of pain that I didn't realize was even there. At times, I was indignant that I had nothing to feel shame about. Even still, I had a lot of shame which was the humiliation I felt. A couple of years went by as I held onto my suffering like a badge of honour, I decided I wasn't spending another moment feeling this way. I de-cluttered my social networks from leftover affiliated acquaintances that really weren't my friends at all and moved on with my head held high. What a relief it was to let that go. I deleted every email I ever sent or received pertaining to this experience and trashed all the administrative files I had kept for posterity's sake. I only kept the good memories and put them out of sight in a box, stored away in my garage.

This experience brought up a lot of suppressed emotion from other negative experiences I have had in the past. It was as though this experience ripped the bandage I had carefully placed over all the pain, discomfort and insecurities I had hidden even from myself.

I began the process of healing through meditation and mindfulness practice. I gave permission and allowed every hurt feeling I ever felt to come to the surface to be released. I had the intention to forgive them and myself. A lot of good work was done. I turned to other counsellors, coaches and energy workers to help me to clean my internal world of thoughts and feelings. Working with others helped me let this go, completely and for good.

The process took almost three years for me to feel at peace. Some may say that is a long time, but it was the time that was necessary for my healing. My commitment to the process brought me through this to the place of forgiveness for others, personal growth and well-being.

"A loving person lives in a loving world. A hostile person lives in a hostile world. Everyone you meet is your mirror."
~ Ken Keyes, Jr. from *Handbook of Higher Consciousness*

Having forgiven others and healed my wounds, something interesting happened to me. I saw the bigger picture as if someone had turned a squeeze-frame into a panoramic scene where everything in that experience was indeed my creation. Like actors playing their parts with seamless portrayal, they knew every line, every movement, and every scene perfectly just as I had scripted. When I was open to letting go of the pain, I was free to see things more clearly.

I realized, I was responsible for everything. I wondered if they would be able to forgive me for the limiting beliefs I held about them. How I judged them to be hurtful and nasty and the way I expected them to treat me with unkindness. How I made poor decisions and took action based on that. I was reactive and defensive. It was me. Like the bottom falling out of a wet paper bag, my story I had told myself collapsed. This is not to say that other people didn't make mistakes, or didn't do anything wrong, or it was my fault, but I acknowledged and took full responsibility for the part I played in creating this reality based on my limiting beliefs, actions and reactions to things. I had to forgive myself. It was time for self-compassion.

Debbie Ford, author of the *Shadow Effect* put it this way, "To allow ourselves to move through our experiences instead of staying stuck in them, we look for how we participated in the circumstances, experiences, and conditions of our lives."

Ask yourself, "What is the gift that this experience holds for me?" I recognize now, in hindsight, that I needed to experience this struggle and the loss of everything for me to do the internal work I needed to do to have everything I have now. I regret nothing. I learned a lot about myself in the process, healed a lot of old wounds and became a stronger person for it. This experience was the accumulation of years of sleepwalking and being a victim of life.

On your journey of transformation, you will come face to face with yourself. All the judgements you've placed on yourself, others, the world, in order to transform your life and shift towards well-being and being well. You will shed the limitations and grow into a vibrant, healthy being who is ready to live life in harmony with love and compassion. This is only possible when healing the negative past, limiting beliefs and you forgive other people and yourself.

You may be considering that you have nothing 'traumatic' to heal. It doesn't have to be traumatic. No matter how insignificant, it can still be healed. Someone cut you off in traffic? Forgive them. Someone said something offensive? Forgive them. You can also forgive yourself for the stories you've told yourself over and over again about such and such who did this and that hurt you, pissed you off, offended you or who just looked at you the wrong way. Remember, forgiveness is the sweetest revenge. The only people you should ever want to get even with are those who have helped you.

Steps to begin the process of forgiveness:

Step 1: Have the intention to forgive. Sometimes this is all you can do—contemplate what forgiveness means.

Step 2: Allow it ALL to be okay in your process to forgive. Intention is the start, but you can begin to activate the healing process. If you are not ready, that is okay. One day you will be ready.

Step 3: Use your imagination to see the light of forgiveness flowing through you and toward the other person. See this light inside of those who you want to forgive. See it being sent back to you with the light of forgiveness shared. If you are forgiving yourself, then imagine your heart opening and light flooding your body. It may be helpful to write a letter of apology to yourself to instigate and let go of the hurt.

Step 4: Repeat whenever you think of that person, the experience or when you need it. Then let it go.

Step 5: When the process of forgiveness is completed you will know. The person or experience will seem as though it is neutral.

How will you know you have forgiven? Forgiveness is feeling as if the wrong had never even occurred. If you find yourself continuing to dwell on the incident or you are resentful or bitter toward the person, even the thought of them causes discomfort, then the process of forgiveness is not complete. If you feel hard done by or you are hard on yourself, they are signs that forgiveness is not yet complete.

If you find yourself in this position, it does not invalidate the steps that you have taken, it simply means that you have not yet arrived at your destination, you just need more time. If you find yourself avoiding situations, places, people, experiences, you know there's good work to be done. Forgiveness is an intentional and active process. It's not words, it is an emotion—it's energetic feelings in motion that come from your heart. You must actively have the intention to forgive until you can honestly look upon the person, or when you think about the person you can do so with compassion.

Brenda J. Bentley

"If you want others to be happy, practice compassion. If you want to be happy, practice compassion."
~ Dalai Lama

Compassion returns you to wholeness. You are what you think about. You are the sum total of your thoughts. Everything that happens to us in life is defined by the meaning you apply to it. No one else defines your experiences. Nothing is good or bad, but your thinking makes it so. It isn't the world that makes you unhappy or the way people are in the world, it's how you process the people and the events in our world.

We don't experience the world as it is, we experience the world as we are. We see the world and others through our own lens. Instead of judging others as people who should be behaving in certain ways, see them as reflecting a part of you and ask yourself "What am I ready to learn from them that will help me to grow?"

Understanding compassion means you understand that everyone suffers, it's an emotion which is essentially empathy. This empathy allows you to reflect on the commonalities between yourself and everyone else. These are the things that make us similar instead of different.

Why develop compassion in your life? Scientific studies suggest there are physical benefits to practicing compassion—people who practice it produce 100 per cent more DHEA, which is a hormone that counteracts the ageing process, and 23 per cent less cortisol—the stress hormone. Dr David Hamilton, author on mind / body / spirit wisdom is clear on how compassion affects you: "When a person shows compassion or kindness it creates an emotional bond between two people, even if it's just short lived. We know from research that when there's a positive emotional bond between people it triggers a release of a hormone called oxytocin in the brain, and also throughout the cardiovascular system, and incredibly oxytocin actually dilates our arteries, and reduces blood pressure because of that. Oxytocin also helps to reduce the levels of inflammation and free radicals in the blood stream—both play a significant role in the geneses of cardiovascular disease."

Here are some steps to practising compassion. Repeat these phrases to yourself often.

Step 1: "Just like me, this person is seeking happiness in his/her life."

Step 2: "Just like me, this person is trying to avoid suffering in his/her life."

Step 3: "Just like me, this person has known sadness, loneliness and despair."

Step 4: "Just like me, this person is seeking to fill his/her needs."

Step 5: "Just like me, this person is learning about life."

Consider that, if you were swimming in the ocean and you encountered a shark and it attacked you would you blame the shark for acting in its nature? Just get out of its way. If someone mistreats you, get out of their way. If you act defensively, you give them something to bounce off of. If you were bitten by a snake, it's not the bite that will kill you; it's the poison it leaves behind. That is what holding onto the pain is doing—poisoning you. Your hurt, sadness, anger, bitterness and resentment come from inside of you and are based on something that happened to you in the past.

When you have removed yourself, feel settled and more detached, reflect on that person who mistreated you. Try to imagine the background of that person. Try to imagine what that person was taught as a child. Try to imagine the day or week that person was going through, and what kind of bad things had happened to that person. Try to imagine the mood and state of mind that person was in—the suffering that person must have been going through to mistreat you that way. And understand that their action was not about you, but about what they were going through. Remember, everyone is doing the best they can at their current level of consciousness and many are sleepwalking.

Now think some more about the suffering of that poor person, and see if you can imagine trying to stop the suffering of that person. And then reflect that if you mistreated someone, and they acted with kindness and compassion toward you, whether that would make you less likely to mistreat that person the next time, and more likely to be kind to that person. Once you have mastered this practice of reflection, try acting with compassion and understanding. Do it in little doses, until you are good at it. Practice makes perfect. Remember, you need to cultivate compassion for yourself and for others to regain peace and well-being in your life.

When it is you that needs forgiveness and compassion the act of self-compassion is needed. Kristen Neff, Associate Professor of Educational Psychology at the University of Austin's definition of self-compassion is: "Being open to and moved by one's own suffering, experiencing feelings of caring and kindness toward oneself, taking an understanding, non-judgemental attitude toward one's inadequacies and failures, and recognizing that one's experience is part of the common human experience."

Being compassionate towards oneself entails recognizing that you did what you could, in that past moment, with what you had at that time. You understand that we all suffer, feel inadequate, make mistakes and have bad judgements. Life experience can be a difficult teacher at times, so it's important to be gentle with ourselves. Everyone experiences difficulties, not everyone has to suffer. However, if you are suffering, being gentle and kind towards yourself will allow you to be more flexible through the growth you gained having experienced this. You remember that being "human" means that one is mortal, vulnerable and imperfect. Therefore, self-compassion means you recognize the universal nature of this human experience through suffering shared.

To practice self-compassion, you can see yourself through the eyes of love. Imagine someone you trust, respect or love and see yourself through their eyes. See what they would see, hear what they would hear, feel how they feel. Imagine they went through what you did. How would they respond to this? Understanding we all hurt at times, it's a universal part of being human. You can take the lessons of this with the perspective of the eyes of love to extend to yourself self-compassion. Take back with you an understanding of reciprocated experience and understanding. Give yourself a break. Give yourself a mental hug. Tell yourself you love yourself for all that you are. You are safe and will grow. Smile. Life is a wonderful series of now moments that you can transform with empowerment of choice. Choose what you really want right now. To move into a vivid, compelling, compassionate life full of blessings you are beaming gratitude for. Leaving the past firmly where it belongs, behind you.

Action Steps:

1. Consider who you need to forgive. Consider forgiving yourself. Consider what it means to forgive.

2. Practice compassion. Remind yourself that everyone is doing the best they can at that time with their current level of consciousness. Use the affirmations "Just like me . . ."

3. Practice self compassion and see yourself through the eyes of love.

Chapter 11—Count Your Blessings

"Be thankful for what you have; you'll end up having more. If you concentrate on what you don't have, you will never, ever have enough."
~ Oprah Winfrey

When I was little, I was taught to always say please and thank you. I was reminded that there were others in this world that didn't have as much as we had, so to be humble and compassionate towards others, and we always began our meals by saying grace. I also attended Catholic school where we began each day with a prayer, followed by one preceding lunch, and then when we returned to set us up for the afternoon lessons, and then again to send us on our way in the evening. It became routine to count our blessings and I'm thankful for that. (See what I did there?)

As I grew up, I experienced many challenges and struggles. What had become a routine way of acknowledging all the good there was in my life through moments of pause and prayer, didn't seem to fit. In fact, I stopped giving thanks all together and started feeling really burdened by life and the cards I had been dealt. Now I was one of those less fortunate people who needed the compassion of other people. It never occurred to me that I should be thankful for the unfortunate times I was experiencing.

If we experience good things in our life, we feel grateful, happy and blessed as a result for the things that happen to us. It's a feeling, emotion, attitude that is cultivated through practice and awareness of what is right in our lives. During our most troublesome experiences, it is the acceptance of what is. It ushers us to look deeper into our pain for the potential for growth and learning. Life becomes our classroom and our experiences our teacher to be grateful for. It is during the darkest of our times, when we hold pain in our hearts and hurt in every cell of our being, broken, confused and bitter that gratitude becomes the beacon of light which shows us the way out.

During the darkest times, remembering to look for the light is the key to moving forward. Those times, when I've wandered away into the shadows becoming despondent, frustrated and dissatisfied with my life's path, when in hindsight I see now they were the road signs, directing me back to love, light and gratitude. It is at these times where I can find the strength inside to give thanks for all that I am given and all that I am learning. Thanks for the teachers, the lessons and the pain.

Changing your perspective about things that happened to you in your life or that are happening takes only the desire to see through the darkness. Clients who have had troubled experiences, resentments and betrayals are taught to look for the deeper blessing of the experience to empower them to see through to the gift of gratitude and healing this will bring.

If you need another reason, then consider how gratitude is good for you. If you have ever met someone who is angry, bitter and resentful, you'll see a person ravaged by their pain. Gratitude heals and rejuvenates the body. At the truest expression, it is energy in motion; emotion that is felt profoundly and deeply. This expression releases endorphins into the bloodstream and not only feels good, but lifts us by enhancing the immune system, which enables the body to resist disease and recover more quickly from illness.

The effect of a grateful outlook on psychological and physical well-being has been examined in a study published in the Journal of Personality and Social Psychology, where participants were randomly assigned experimental conditions such as hassles, gratitude listing and either neutral life events or social comparison, and kept records of their moods, coping behaviors, health behaviors, physical symptoms, and overall life appraisals. Findings suggest that when participants focussed on blessings they were 25% happier than those who didn't.

How can you practice being more grateful? Here are some ideas:

- **Gratitude Journal**—Establish a daily practice to remind yourself of the gifts, benefits and things you enjoy. Make it part of your daily routine to write down at least three things you are grateful or happy about. It doesn't have to be anything monumental; it can be a sunny sky, smile of someone you love, the playfulness of your pet, birdsong or anything that makes you smile. It can be something that went well for you today or something associated with ordinary events or people.
- **Remember the Struggles**—Hindsight provides the potential for reflection on how far you've come from where you have been before, during hard or painful experiences, giving you contrast to examine differences which make the difference.
- **Affirm I am**—Through external reminders such as photographs, pictures, paintings, quotes or your own personal affirmations, you can affirm and reaffirm "I am grateful" and your language can reflect this with using words and symbolism that remind you of the blessings, fortune, abundance and prosperity in your life.
- **Say Thank You**—Kindness is contagious and you can share this with others by always saying "thank you" even if it's the smallest of gestures.
- **Random Acts of Kindness**—Smile and the world smiles back. Test it and prove to yourself that you can invite

others into your feelings of gratefulness by invoking in them the emotion by the simple act of smiling for no reason at all. People may wonder what your secret is, and this may make you smile even more to know it's just to be grateful and to shine your light into the world.

- **Practice Heartfelt Gratitude**—First thing in the morning and last thing before you go to sleep at night, imagine at least five things you can be aware of that you are grateful for. They can be big or small things. Picture them in your mind. Imagine sending love from your heart to that thing, person or experience. Allow this heartfelt gratitude to swell and expand inside of you and like a light allow it to flow from you out into the world, smoothing the way for every experience you've had and that you are going to have. You can also practice this when faced in any challenge or difficulty. You may not understand yet the relevance or reward of wisdom this challenge will gift you with, so send the loving energy or heartfelt gratitude shining from you toward the person or experience that is challenging. You will feel more at peace and whatever the difficulty, you'll be able to deal with it from a place of kindness and love.

Practiced, you will feel happier and more contented in your life. Blended together with being more present minded, forgiving yourself and others, using your imagination in a powerful and positive way, and letting go of limiting beliefs and affirming supporting ones, you can create the experience of life you want. Create a fulfilled life, full of love and enjoying more things in your life to be grateful for. It is the essence of gratefulness that you attract more things to be grateful for.

Action Points:

1. Practice being grateful for everything throughout your day.

2. Notice how much better you feel to appreciate all that life is.

Eat, Guilt, Repent, Repeat

I asked for strength and
God gave me difficulties to make me strong.

I asked for wisdom and
God gave me problems to solve.

I asked for prosperity and
God gave me brawn and brains to work.

I asked for courage and
God gave me dangers to overcome.

I asked for patience and
God placed me in situations where I was forced to wait.

I asked for love and
God gave me troubled people to help.

I asked for favours and
God gave me opportunities.

I received nothing I wanted
I received everything I needed.

My prayers have all been answered.

Author Unknown

Chapter 12—Manage Your Emotions, Without Food

"Feelings are meant to be felt—not fed!"
~ Brenda Bentley

The above quote is one I repeat every day to my clients who are emotional eaters. Are you an emotional eater? Answer the questions below:

Does your hunger come on suddenly and you feel you need to eat NOW?

Does you hunger feel urgent?

Do you crave specific foods at certain times of day?

Do you feel guilty after eating?

Do you eat mindlessly or when you are distracted?

Do you eat past the point of fullness?

Do you obsess about food?

Do you feel you need to treat yourself?

Do you feel compelled to eat food?

Do you feel hollow or empty inside and use food to fill you up?

Do you feel that food calms you down?

Do you feel food protects you from feeling things in some way?

You probably already have a good idea that you have limiting behaviors, beliefs and conditioning that has developed into a poor relationship with food. This chapter is to give you strategies for managing your emotional state without food. What you have discovered is that weight loss is really about self-esteem, which means there are changes to your psychological and emotional connection to yourself, and food has to happen if you're going to be successful long term. If you think that just changing your diet and exercise habits will give the results you want in the long run, then you are fooling yourself. The mental breakthrough is necessary and at the core of this transformation is applying new ways of managing your thoughts, feelings and behaviors. Emotions are very powerful and can be destructive and a little bit of negativity can kill your dream. Managing your emotions is an important life skill to learn.

Our emotions act as a feedback system—our emotional navigational system or GPS. They navigate us to let us know when we are heading towards what we want or away from what we want. Sometimes our feelings start with a thought, sometimes it seems our feelings start and create thoughts, the point is they are both closely related to one another and it is hard to tell them apart at times. By learning to live consciously and be aware, you are empowered to have control over your thoughts, feelings and behaviors. This will give you the experience of the life you want, but takes a little bit of practice. It's a life skill.

Whenever you feel bad . . . upset . . . anxious . . . fearful, you can be sure that you are thinking about something you do not want—that you want to avoid—or not have / feel. Our thoughts feel like they happen to us and we have no control over them, our thoughts are spontaneous, but you now know more than ever that you do have control over what you think and with practice you can exercise great control over how you feel.

Many of my clients feel too much. They feel their emotions, other people's emotions and they are at times confused as to whether their feelings are even their own. This confusion leads them to turn to food for comfort. Emotional eating only masks the feeling temporarily. The feeling will be there after the binge, but will have a layer of guilt on top. You've already come to learn that by taking responsibility for your thoughts and feelings that you can be aware of when you are absorbing the emotional energy of others. It's important to recognize you always have a choice. It's a good thing to be sensitive! It has taken me years to recognize that my emotional sensitivity is not a curse, it is a blessing. I am in touch with my feelings and the feelings of others, but I do not have to absorb or experience anything I do not wish to, just by remembering one thing: Do I want to feel this way or not? If you do not want to feel that way, then you remove yourself from the situation or person that is draining you.

Most problems exist because we do not want to accept the way things are. You resist it. You block it. You suppress it—push it down. Sometimes you express it—get angry or frustrated about it. There is another choice and it's learning how to release.

When we grow up, due to social, cultural, family influences and factors, we learn to suppress our emotions. You can see how children, in their natural state before this conditioning are very good at expressing their emotions—also releasing these emotions.

What is releasing then? You've seen children playing, or you remember when you were little yourself, running around on the playground, then fall down, hurt themselves and they look around to see if anyone is looking . . . If they have a suitable audience, then they may cry for some attention or run over, to have it looked at and 'kissed better'. Once they have what they need, they let it go . . . naturally—and get right back to playing! Children naturally release unwanted emotions. It's only as we grow up and we are told it's not okay to express, that we learn to suppress. Suppression becomes the most natural thing to do . . . but it's also the most harmful to our well-being.

How do you re-learn how to release?

As I mentioned, resisting or blocking is the main reason that you hold onto unwanted emotions. It may sound paradoxical, but by resisting the way you are feeling, you keep it in place: even if you are not ready to 'let it go' because you're still mad / sad / hurt / angry / upset.

The cure is to feel free to resist, it eliminates itself. I often ask clients to 'watch themselves with curiosity' as if they were going to write a research paper on how they do their problem. When you find yourself resisting something instead, just watch; notice how you are doing the problem. Give yourself permission to feel whatever you are feeling. Be present with the feeling. Let it be what it is—without judgement, without wanting to stop feeling that way. Trying to stop resisting is just more resisting, and then when you stop trying to stop trying to resist you add another layer, and it just goes on and on.

How to Release Emotion

How are you feeling? Take a moment of reflection and tune into what you are feeling in your body. Below are the steps to take to release anything you are not wanting to feel, and you are not willing to continue to feel anymore. Ask yourself:

Do I want to continue to feel like this? YES / NO

If YES—then that's great, let it be okay you choose to feel this way!

Could I allow myself to feel everything I needed to feel about this? YES / NO

Whatever you are feeling, could you love or appreciate the feeling exactly as it is? YES / NO

If not, could you love or appreciate yourself for feeling the feeling? YES / NO

If not, could you love or appreciate yourself for not being willing or able to love or appreciate yourself for feeling the feeling? YES / NO

If not, could you find another aspect of whatever you are experiencing until you are feeling a genuine sense of love or appreciation for yourself or the feeling? YES / NO

Now ask yourself:

Could you let go and release this feeling? YES / NO

If yes, can you release it now? YES / NO

If not, when can you release it? (Later, after I'm done feeling it.)

If not, what is the one thing you need to learn before you can release this feeling for good?

Remember you may not be able to understand fully WHY you are feeling this way and would it change how you're feeling if you did? Probably not. Let go of your need to analyze and understand why. Instead, focus on what you can learn from this feeling.

The purpose is to let and allow yourself to feel whatever it is you need to feel and let it be okay. That doesn't mean you have to be happy about it or you approve of what happened to upset you. What it means is that you, when you are ready, can return to your balanced, natural, default place of neutrality and move on. Your emotions are like a navigation system—they are telling you that you need to learn something about the situation so you can grow and get back on course to where you want to be.

Loving Your Feelings

A great 'in the moment' strategy for dealing with negative emotions is to love them away. This is not because you love feeling bad or you love pain, it's because you know that your emotions have a purpose and you are courageous enough to give yourself permission to be fully present with your feelings. This will not overwhelm you, it will make you stronger. It also gives you power over the emotion so you can transcend it.

Step 1: Whatever you are feeling—name it: "I am feeling *afraid*."

Step 2: Feel that feeling inside your body.

Step 3: Imagine pushing this feeling out in front of you and notice how it represents itself.

Step 4: Imagine you can step right inside of that feeling courageously. Scream at it, "Bring it on! I love being *afraid*!" (or whatever your feeling is)

Step 5: Repeat Step 4 until you feel the intensity of the feeling has passed and you've come out the other side of it. In this place, you should feel peaceful.

By giving yourself permission and releasing negative feelings you reset your body to balanced state. Suppressed emotions can cause disease in the body. All challenges / difficulties we face in our lives are only opportunities to learn something about ourselves and how we can love ourselves even more.

It's okay to feel emotions. Feelings are meant to be felt, not fed. By attempting to feed your emotions, you are dumping them into a void inside that can never change how you feel, except by adding to that feeling with another layer of guilt, shame or numbness.

Action Steps:

1. Understand that your feelings are important feedback.

2. When you are feeling an emotion, don't turn to food, use the strategies detailed here.

3. Learn to release and practice it so you can do so whenever you need to.

4. Learn to love your feelings away and practice it so you can do this whenever you need to.

5. Once feeling peaceful, you can objectively evaluate your hunger.

Chapter 13—Eating Intuitively

"The intuitive mind is a sacred gift and the rational mind is a faithful servant. We have created a society that honours the servant and has forgotten the gift."
~ Albert Einstein

At this point, we are bringing together all the differences which will make the difference as you begin to heal the relationships with yourself, your past, your beliefs, and begin to use your mind positively, productively and supportively, moving you towards your transformation. Here we are at the place where you can now take all the ideas, experiments, strategies, concepts, exercises and move forward so you can break the cycle permanently and change direction to well-being and being well.

The term Intuitive Eating was created by Evelyn Tribole and Elyse Resch. Both are registered dieticians in California who after years of trying to help their patients with structured eating plans that failed, decided to work together to write the book *Intuitive Eating: A Revolutionary Program That Really Works*. In the book, which I consider the bible on the approach is the 10 Principles of Intuitive Eating. Below are the principles I've adapted:

1. Reject the Diet Mentality. As you discovered in earlier chapters, dieting doesn't work. By rejecting the diet mentality you get back in rapport with yourself so you can honour your biological hunger and give yourself the gift of trust. You have all the internal wisdom you need to know how to eat and when to stop when you are comfortably satisfied. You have forgotten how to do this through years of following dieting rules. Diets offer the empty promise of weight loss but the effects are temporary. Focus on creating meaningful and lasting change by developing trust of yourself, love and acceptance for your body and managing your emotional state in a healthy and productive way. This is the difference that makes the difference and will give you more happiness and fulfilment in your life that really matters.

It may take some time for you to get out of the dieting mentality. You've spent years learning how to eat based on rules. Be patient with yourself and understand that getting back in touch with your body is a process. The most important thing to do is to consider that you can stop dieting from here on out.

2. Honour Your Hunger. Are you hungry? Do you know what it feels like to be hungry? You can develop a sensitivity of your physical hunger cues so you can respond and be certain that you are giving your body the nutrition and respect necessary for you to return to your default, healthy natural weight. You cannot outwit your biology. Your body's autonomy will assert itself above anything you attempt to do. Listen, hear, understand and respond and reward your hunger cues to reinforce and make you more sensitive to the many different ways hunger speaks to you.

You may not even recognize hunger. It may be you've spent years being hungry and staving yourself with diets. Being able to recognize hunger is a skill. Like any new skill you need to practice it. It starts every morning when you wake up and you break your fast. From there you can begin to wait until you notice how your body communicates hunger to you. Approach this learning with curiosity.

3. Make Peace with Food. Guilt is no longer on the menu! By giving yourself unconditional permission to eat whatever you want, you are removing the need to feel guilty. It may be quite a scary prospect to do this as you may think you're going to be out of control around food. Studies show that when we allow access to all types of foods, habituation takes place. Which simply means, if you have it, you don't want it as much as you would if you couldn't have it. By ditching the rule-based and fear-based agendas in this process you will be empowering yourself with choice. Restriction and deprivation gives food power over you. Real choice is in whatever you really want, not what you think you should be eating or when you think you should be eating it. It is good and right that you enjoy the food you eat to the utmost. This liberates you and food becomes less seductive. When food becomes a neutral and balanced approach to your eating, your real preferences will begin to shine through. This means that you may be surprised that all the forbidden foods you crave, desire and wanted, just have lost their allure.

In the process you will be making all foods emotionally neutral and free from conditions. That means you can experiment with your forbidden foods and really discover what your preferences are when you strip away the rule and fear based agendas around food. You will need to remind yourself often that you can have whatever you want to eat. There should be no food that is off limits. As you get in rapport with your body, you will be able to hear what your preferences are and this will not be based on what you think you should eat.

4. Challenge the Food Police. Be aware that there are a lot of people in this world who are still following diets and they probably will until they too hit diet bottom and wake-up to the reality that diets don't work. In this process, many people will tell you, share with you advice and provide you with guidance. You will see it on television, read about it in magazines but you are now armed with the ability of choice to understand and know that this change is an inside job. You can just smile, nod or get on your soapbox and scream out to the world that there is another way and this way has absolutely nothing really to do with food restriction, calorie counting, point systems or other food-based rules.

People will not understand that you are not on a diet. This is what they think works right now and they have not hit diet bottom. They may be someone who has never struggled with their weight. People will tell you that you can't eat certain foods. Let it be okay. When they begin to see the difference in you and as your body changes, they will leave you to it.

5. Respect Your Fullness. Biological hunger can be satisfied in only one way: with food. As you learn how much is enough for you, through being aware of the sensory cues, and training yourself to know that you are ready to begin to stop eating because you've all that your body requires to feel comfortably full. This will shift your emphasis on the importance of focussing on how your body feels when you eat certain foods.

You may be eating until you are full up. There is a difference between fullness and satisfaction. You can never feel satisfied if you are eating for emotional reasons. What you are hungry for isn't food.

6. Discover the Satisfaction Factor. Eating is one of our most basic survival instincts and like all life sustaining instincts such as eating and sex, it's supposed to be pleasurable! When you eat what you really want and take the time to enjoy it, you will experience the satisfaction and pleasure you've probably been missing. This pleasure principle means you feel more fulfilled and can be satisfied with much less than before.

7. Honour Your Feelings Without Using Food. Feelings are meant to be felt, not fed. Learn new ways to provide self care and manage your feelings in a way that supports your transformation. Emotions are no longer on the menu! As you learn and apply the strategies for managing uncomfortable emotions you learn in this book, you will be empowered to no longer be reactive to your environment. You will be creative and in the position to choose how you want to feel or feel how you feel without suffering over it.

8. Respect Your Body. Your body has supported you throughout your lifetime, even if it has limitations. By respecting your body you learn to dismiss media promoted ideas of perfection and honour your default, healthy non-dieting weight that is right for you. We are not one-size-fits all and come in a variety of shapes, heights, weights, structures and figures. It's important to accept this as a fact and stop chasing the illusion. We all know that glossy magazines are airbrushed, celebrities can afford time to work out all day long and get surgical enhancements, but we still think this is the right way and our bodies are wrong. In order to totally reject the diet mentality you need to be realistic, loving and accepting about your body just as it is and it will support you in your transformation to a healthy weight, size and shape that's right for you. By not doing so it's like you are 5'10" tall and want to be 5'2"—you can try and try, but the reality is you are 5'10"! Body acceptance means you can love your way to the healthy size that's right for you. Your body has an inherent wisdom that you can begin to respect more.

9. Exercise and Feel the Difference. Focus on how things feel and the benefits when you consider movement. Personally, I prefer to use the word 'movement' instead of 'exercise' as so much of what we do is exercise through movement! Also, when we focus on how we feel after we've been active and the benefits of doing so, it motivates us so much more than thinking you need to do it because you ate that donut yesterday. What you do consistently matters, even if it's 15 minutes each day.

10. Honour Your Health—Gentle Nutrition. It's not the occasional slice of cake that makes us fat. It's what we do consistently that matters. When you are returning to eating intuitively, you will go through a phase of introducing back into your world all the forbidden foods you were once deprived, which is very important in allowing your preferences to shine through. Once you've habituated and make food neutral, you will begin to recognize your preferences. By honouring and respecting your health you recognize that you do not have to be perfect in all the choices you make to be healthy.

As you learn to return to eating intuitively, embracing your health, returning to well-being by rejecting old conditioning you've learned from diets, you will open up to a whole new way to experience eating.

In a super size culture where there is a vast array of choice, convenience and portion sizes that would make a heavyweight boxer groan, it's understandable how our trust in ourselves has eroded. You may have told yourself that eating fatty foods that are high in calories are addictive. Food production is a business and yes, they do want you to eat their brand of food so they can make profit. When you learn to incorporate eating intuitively and mindfully after healing your relationships with food, and you can understand that you are 100% responsible for what goes into your mouth there is no need to stress or worry about it anymore.

Did you know that Americans worry about food more than any other culture in the world? This worry and stress creates an unhealthy relationship with food which is apparent when you compare it to other cultures and their eating philosophies. Take for instance the French and Japanese. The French love their bread, butter, croissants, pâté, wine and cheese! They eat the richest food types in Europe but are also the slimmest, naturally. The French essentially are able to eat three times as much fat as Americans but are slimmer and have a lower incidence of heart disease.

The key is mindful eating practice where they eat less, but enjoy it more intensely. By comparison, an American serving size is 25% to 75% larger depending on the restaurant (such as all you can eat establishments) than in France.

It really comes down to quality versus quantity. What this shows is the choice to eat a lot of food for a bargain price or to eat based on quality of the food, experience and taste. I guess you will need to consider when making a decision whether you are happy where you are, at the size you are and with your current eating habits. If you consider the full price you are paying for eating the way you are, those $2 for 2 hamburgers are really not a bargain to your health after all.

By tuning into your body and your preferences to eat what you really want to eat then you can make a choice based on that. Slow down your eating and take a moment to pause throughout your meal to feel how full you are. Knowing that you can always take home any leftovers and eat it again when you are hungry, if that is in fact what you fancy eating—and talk about bargains, that could be tomorrow's lunch in the doggy bag! You will feel tempted all the time if you are restricting or depriving yourself, so remember to give yourself unconditional permission to eat what you want.

Like the French, in Japan their experience of eating is to be savoured. It is customary that meal times take two hours or more. The whole process including preparing, takes much longer than that. You may be thinking you don't have time for any of that as you are already so busy and this may be true. If you feel as though you are thinly stretched across the demands of your life, your career, your kids, your household responsibilities and haven't even got time for eating then this is really not a question of eating mindfully, it's about a life change.

Sure, we all feel stretched at times and have too much on our plate (in both ways!). However, you must realize that if you were to look back on your life, having made the choices you have, to push yourself to the brink of unhappiness and despair that you cannot take time to sit, eat, enjoy the experience of eating your food, then what is living for?

In her bestselling book, *French Women Don't Get Fat*, Mireille Guiliano says the French lifestyle is "more than a list of habits in isolation—it is a total mindset." The experience is about putting time into preparation and the enjoyment of the process of it all. You browse the market and buy seasonal fruits and vegetables, carefully picking them out by their smell and feel. All day long, you anticipate eating that perfectly ripe pear or ideally green asparagus. Once it's time to eat, you savour every mouthful. Guiliano recalls her mother enjoying one chocolate a day as if it were a religious experience. She also advises you to eat about half of what you think you want to eat. At which time you can evaluate your hunger and fullness levels.

Research shows that our experience of eating food is multi-sensory experience which means we see, hear, smell, taste and feel the food we eat. We are stimulated on many levels and when we take the time to allow ourselves to be stimulated fully, we get more satisfaction and more pleasure. Remember, at the end of your life, looking back, you will not remember missing the American Idol final on television but you will remember one of the best meals of your life you took the time to share and enjoy fully.

It is said that it takes between 15 and 20 minutes for food you eat to reach the first part of the small intestine which sends a chemical signal back to the brain to say "no longer hungry." In this fast-paced world, we eat on the go, when multi-tasking or unconsciously, and when we eat too fast, we can easily put too much food into our bodies before the satiety signals are received. When you feed your biological hunger and take the time to eat slowly and savour each mouthful, you can pay attention to all the textures on a multi-sensory level. You can notice the subtle difference between the first mouthful which was probably experienced with intense flavour and that of the fifth or sixth mouthful when the sensations decrease as hunger goes to being neutral.

The French and Japanese have a lot you can learn from in their approach to eating. By focussing on your preferences, enjoying the process, preparation and anticipation of eating foods that you can take time out to share and enjoy, the whole experience will be so much more pleasurable it will be easy to leave food when you recognize the feeling of satiety and can say "I am no longer hungry."

As you are discovering being present in the moment, being mindful of your thoughts, feelings and behaviors, you will experience a powerful shift in the way you've been running your life up to now. It will bring you remarkable, amazing and powerful changes to being a conscious creator of life. Part of this positive change is about learning to eat mindfully.

Principles of Mindful Eating has been thoughtfully outlined by The Centre For Mindful Eating:

Principles of Mindfulness:

- Mindfulness is deliberately paying attention with non-judgmental awareness
- Mindfulness encompasses both internal processes and external environments

- Mindfulness is being aware of what is present for you mentally, emotionally and physically in each moment.
- With practice, mindfulness cultivates the possibility of freeing yourself of reactive, habitual patterns of thinking, feeling and acting
- Mindfulness promotes balance, choice, wisdom and acceptance of what is

Mindful Eating is:

- Allowing yourself to become aware of the positive and nurturing opportunities that are available through food preparation and consumption by respecting your own inner wisdom
- Choosing to eat food that is both pleasing to you and nourishing to your body by using all your senses to explore, savour and taste
- Acknowledging responses to food (likes, neutral or dislikes) without judgment
- Learning to be aware of physical hunger and satiety cues to guide your decision to begin eating and to stop eating

Someone Who Eats Mindfully:

- Acknowledges that there is no right or wrong way to eat but there are varying degrees of awareness surrounding the experience of food
- Accepts that his/her eating experiences are unique
- Is an individual who by choice, directs his/her awareness to all aspects of food and eating on a moment-by-moment basis
- Is an individual who looks at the immediate choices and direct experiences associated with food and eating: not to the distant health outcome of that choice

- Is aware of and reflects on the effects caused by unmindful eating
- Experiences insight about how he/she can act to achieve specific health goals as he/she becomes more attuned to the direct experience of eating and feelings of health
- Becomes aware of the interconnection of earth, living beings, and cultural practices and the impact his/her food choices have on those systems

There are multi-sensory ways you experience hunger as stimulated and understood through our cognitions, which are:

- Eyes (sight of food)
- Nose (smell of food)
- Tongue (taste of food)
- Touch (feel of food in our mouth)
- Sound (noise of food being prepared and eating)
- Mind
- Thoughts
- Feelings
- Memories
- Concept of Self

Physical Hunger

- Hunger pangs or gnawing feeling
- Emptiness
- Sickly feeling
- Dizziness
- Agitation
- Headache
- Fatigue
- Difficulty concentrating

The differences between physical and emotional hunger from Brian Wansink's book *Mindless Eating* are that physical hunger builds gradually, is felt physically in the body, goes away after eating whereas emotional hunger is sudden and urgent, is not felt but understood in the mind and is unrelated to time or physical sensations.

When food is before us, we might experience sensory hunger. Jan Chozen Bays, M.D., has described different types of hunger in her book *Mindful Eating*.

- **Hunger:** This is what the eye sees—now listen to what the mind says
- **Hunger:** Smell—now listen to what the mind says
- **Hunger:** Is your mouth hungry?—now listen to what the mind says
- **Hunger:** Notice if the stomach is full or not, satisfied or not, after you take a bite.

Everyone has had the experience of gulping down their food while multi-tasking or eating mindlessly and then got that sudden surprise when there's no more food on their plate. In the book *The Slow Down Diet: Eating For Pleasure, Energy, And Weight Loss* by Marc David it states that "the brain must experience taste, pleasure, aroma, and satisfaction so it can accurately assess a meal and catalyze our most efficient digestive force. When we eat too fast or fail to notice our food, the brain interprets this missed experience as hunger."

This means that your mind won't register your eating experience fully and this could lead to overeating. In order to experience the most satisfaction, you need to slow down and be fully aware of the process.

There is also **Practical Hunger**. Practical hunger happens when you know you will not be able to eat so you eat outside of hunger as it's practical to do so. The most important thing about eating intuitively is you know yourself well enough to make choices that will support your health and feel good to you. For example, I had to travel to London to deliver a seminar and knew I wouldn't be able to eat when I became hungry. I wasn't hungry when I set out on my travels that day, as I had already had breakfast, but I ate lunch early and quite a lot of it in fact. I ate for practical reasons as I knew it would be a good six hours until I was able to eat again and there would be no access to snacking foods to get me through.

I managed to get through the whole seminar comfortably and by dinner time, I was hungry again, so I ate. Eating intuitively is about flexibility and honoring your health. You are the expert of you and you will learn to trust your instincts to know what is best for you.

Sometimes we hunger for something that isn't related to food. When this happens, it is helpful to pause and ask yourself, "What am I really hungry for?" Allow yourself to think beyond food. When you do this, you can begin to include some other needs you hunger for. The work by Marshall Rosenberg, Ph.D., called *Non-Violent Communication*, acknowledges that every person has some basic needs. These include:

- Meaning and Purpose
- Autonomy (independence)
- Safety
- Empathy
- Sustenance (food, nourishment for body, mind and spirit)
- Creativity
- Love
- Community
- Rest/Relax/Play

Being mindful about your emotional and psychological needs will develop with your awareness and make the clear distinction between genuine, physical hunger, emotional hunger and sensory hunger. There are no rules to eating intuitively and mindfully, except to say that you are aware and you are paying attention to how you are thinking, feeling and acting about food.

You can develop your awareness by using the hunger scales and charts below of common feelings that arise to help us know if a need is or is not being met. A copy of this is available for download from the website at www.eatguiltrepentrepeat. com so whenever you think about food you can refer to this scale to retrain yourself and become attuned with your body's signals again. You may consider placing a copy of this on your refrigerator someplace predominant so you can refer to it with ease.

The Hunger Scale	Guidelines
1—Physically faint	Eat whenever you're hungry
2—Ravenous	
3—Hungry	Eat what you want, not what you think you should
4—Peckish	
5—Neutral	Eat consciously and enjoy every mouthful
6—Pleasantly satisfied	
7—Full	Stop when you think you're full
8—Stuffed	**Remember!**
9—Bloated	Emotional hunger is sudden and urgent; physical hunger is gradual and patient. Emotional hunger cannot be satisfied with food; physical hunger can. Check you may be thirsty. The signal for hunger is the same as for thirst. Have a glass of water and then wait 5-10 minutes to see if you're still hungry. Pause halfway through your meal and check-in with yourself. Close your eyes and feel your fullness. Take your time. Remember, it takes 15-20 minutes for the brain to register fullness.
10—Nauseous	

Mindful eating takes practice. Like any new skill, you need to do it repeatedly before it becomes second nature.

Action Points:

1. Use the hunger scales to retrain yourself to know when you are hungry and satisfied.

2. Aim to eat when you are at a 3 or 4 and stop eating when you are at 5 or 6.

3. Follow the Principles for Intuitive Eating—you can download a copy from the website.

4. Eat mindfully with full awareness and slow down to enjoy your meals.

Chapter 14—The Feeling of Movement

"The secret of getting ahead is getting started."
~ Mark Twain

A lot of emphasis has been placed on the mind in this book and how our thoughts affect how we feel and our body. We've explored our belief systems and how these can shape our bodies and get in the way of us achieving what we want for ourselves. Most people understand that exercise and getting active is an important part of a healthy lifestyle, but a lot of people struggle with maintaining any form of regular activity. Some people think that exercise is only about weight loss or weight control and miss the fact that health and well-being affect both mind and body and are essential for optimal healthy lifestyle.

A lot of limiting thoughts and beliefs surround exercising and being active—and here are some typical ones to help you build a more positive and resourceful attitude toward movement and motivation for exercise.

"I know I should exercise but I hate it so I have to make myself do it." Examine the previous statement and you'll find negative beliefs and attitudes built in with words such as *should* and *hate* and *make myself*. These beliefs and attitudes are born out of previous experiences and meanings attached to them whether this comes from boredom experienced during exercise routines, discomfort or pain developed, not being chosen for teams or having difficulties in school that were connected to gym / physical fitness / PE. All of these create negative emotional and psychological connections to exercise.

Exercise often becomes a punishment for overeating as some people only ever take up exercise when they have the goal of slimming. The more you can make the prospect of physical activity fun and part of your lifestyle the more likely it will become a healthy habit. Research proves that little and often is better than big chunks so you can start off slowly in small amounts of time (even if it's 5 minutes here, 10 minutes there) and build up gradually to something that fits in with you. It's important that you focus your mind on the benefits that being more active will bring you—like how wonderful you will feel instead of how much weight you *should* lose.

"I don't have time." The truth is everyone has time; they just spend their time on other activities they perceive as being more pressing or more important. The average person watches over two hours of television each day. I can confidently say you will never regret missing *The Bachelor* more than you will miss feeling healthy, happy and well when you are not. If you make it a part of your lifestyle, routine and fun, you will look forward to the time you spend in this way, because you will know that it makes you feel good.

"I don't have the energy." It is a catch 22 cycle that you may not feel you have the energy right now as you perceive the monumental task of taking on a new exercise regime because you need to lose weight. In fact, just by thinking about it in this way will be about using willpower for you to choose to exercise over watching television, and it will seem daunting when you first start out. The truth is that gentle but consistent exercise increases feelings of well-being minutes after starting to exercise. Exercise increases strength and stamina so you can sleep better, making you more productive and more energetic in all you do. The key is to say yes when you have a choice to do something. The positive attitude you gain toward taking action comes from focussing on the benefits of taking action. Focus on how much energy you'll have and how good you'll feel. It is also important that you *could* do this, which is about capability—and you are capable to go for a gentle walk at lunch aren't you? And you *would* do this, which is about willingness because you know the benefits it will bring. But should you? Delete this word from your vocabulary. Should implies you are being forced and taking positive action in your life means you are creating positive change in your life. Positive action leads to more positive action as positive results stack together, making it easy to just do it.

So much of what you do in a day takes energy. Breathing takes energy! You burn calories when you are sleeping! Once you've applied the learning shared in this book and you are eating normally you will have healed your metabolism from its P.T.D.D. (post traumatic dieting disorder - *not an actual diagnosis!*), your body will begin to burn off excess energy stored. Consider all the things you do every day that burn energy. For example, one hour worth of housework can burn approximately 300 calories! In this process, you can come to appreciate that by feeding yourself real food, in moderate amounts, moving your body, feeling good in yourself is the most healthy and natural way to achieve a healthy weight that is right for you.

The biggest hurdle to overcome is your mind. What other negative thoughts, beliefs and attitudes do you hold about being active? Refer back on the chapter on dismantling limiting beliefs so you can focus on what you can do. Remember, what you focus on with your thoughts and your inner dialogue has an effect on you. Learn to develop a positive mindset and use the tools provided here to create resourceful beliefs that support your transformation.

You can shift your thoughts to something more resourceful, so instead of saying "exercise is boring" say "being active fills my body with energy and feel good chemicals" or "I'm going to sleep better than ever after this workout!" or "every step I take towards where I want to go is success." Think about yourself as a healthy and active person and you will become one. Think and repeat "I am active and radiating health, I am." Prove to yourself what a difference it makes to you in your life!

To help you to develop this positive mindset use the *Movement & Motivation for Exercise* self hypnosis MP3 available with the companion workbook and audio toolkit from the website.

Action Steps:

1. Focus on the benefits of movement.

2. Just say YES when you would have said no and move your body because it feels good.

3. Consider all that you do each day that burns stored energy.

4. Dismantle any limiting beliefs you have been telling yourself.

5. Repeat new healthy affirmations that empower you.

6. You may consider downloading the audio tool for Movement and Motivation from www. eatguiltrepentrepeat.com

Chapter 15—Practice Makes Permanent

"Our life is an apprenticeship to the truth that around every circle another can be drawn; that there is no end in nature, but every end is a beginning, and under every deep a lower deep opens."
~ Ralph Waldo Emerson

Putting this philosophy into action with all the other lessons involved in this book will mean you take the time to learn, understand, practice and apply them into your life. So far, we've explored how your thoughts affect your feelings and your behaviors. How your beliefs affect your biology, your perception, actions/reactions and are a fundamental part of shaping your perception of reality. We've also explored how to create a successful intention and creation goal statement that will produce real results step-by-step. We've explored present moment awareness and how to get as much enjoyment out of eating as humanly possible!

It's a lot to take on board. Let it be okay that there is a learning curve to all of this. By taking each step and working through the process, at your own pace, you will get there. This process is a proven way to transform yourself for meaningful and lasting change, without dieting. Remember, change is a process and practice makes permanent. The more you do it the easier it gets!

Creating Fulfilment

"The more intensely we feel about an idea or a goal, the more assuredly the idea, buried deep in our subconscious, will direct us along the path to its fulfilment."
~ Earl Nightingale, American author and motivational speaker

What if you already knew that your life would be happy and fulfilled by the thoughts, feelings, decisions, choices and actions you've made. How much easier would it be for you to face any of life's challenges from this point on?

If you were to imagine stretching out before your whole future and all the experiences you are to have along the way, all the way, to the end of your long and fulfilled life to that very moment you could imagine looking back as the older, wiser person you are in the future, sitting, resting in your rocking chair, satisfied with the life you have created, the experiences you've had and shared and what you have achieved, how much easier would this be for you? To really allow the wonder of knowing and deep contentment for the life you have lived and be the person you are. What you've overcome, you've learned and grown from. The blessings you can count and what you believe about yourself, your capabilities and abilities. All those things that are important to you that expand the gift of having lived this life to your fullest potential and shared it with those you love.

To spend as much time as you need to understand and absorb the qualities, feelings and sense for this to be aware, in your own time and your own way to let go and trust that everything will be perfectly experienced. You've lived the life you wanted the way you wanted and you can bring back the subtle guidance, insights and understandings that in this future you just know, to lead you to that you, you know you are becoming, just waiting for you in the future, your fulfilled life. How good it will be to begin to let this unfold in the perfect order of all things, let it be just as it is. So you can begin to recognize on many levels the differences this makes to you now, to know that from today you are living and creating the fulfilled life you know is waiting for you, there in the future, in direct proportion to your ability to vividly see it, feel it, know it and trust that it is there as already accomplished.

Bringing to your awareness now possibilities and potentials that take you towards the future you. So whatever the next thing is that lets you know this is happening, your life changing towards the direction of your desire and how this changes the way you act and react to everything around you—we can both be curious. So whether it happens now or later, it doesn't matter, it's only important that it does happen. Which means you can just relax and let go on this journey toward your highest potential and greatest fulfilment, and every challenge is just another opportunity to learn, grow and overcome, creating the future you, right now.

With your journey to this point so far, you've learned how to unlock and release all you need to within you and without you to move forward and consider this transformation you've already begun as you fill your thoughts with these empowering words.

Action Steps:

1. Imagine the possibilities!

2. The more you focus your mind and improve the quality of your consciousness the happier you will be. The happier you feel the easier it is to repeat behaviors that support your transformation.

Chapter 16—Commitment Contract

"Stay committed to your decisions, but stay flexible in your approach."
~ Tom Robbins

Begin your journey of transformation by creating a contract with yourself. Once you have resolved and released anything that is potentially standing in your way of making positive change, consider this contract bound by self trust. This contract will remind you of the priorities in the transformative process and reinforce your commitment to change.

I agree to nourish myself when I am hungry.

I agree to acknowledge that change is a process and there are high and low points.

I agree to lean into the process of change and get out of my own way so it's easier.

I agree to focus on how I feel in all things, not how it looks.

I agree to learn to love and accept myself as I am.

I agree to switch negative thoughts to positive, supporting thoughts.

I agree to take with a pinch of salt, advice from food police, chronic dieters and critics.

I agree to focus on movement as a way to feel good within myself.

I agree that I will meet my basic essential needs, whatever that means to me.

I agree to pamper myself and have quality 'me time', whatever that means to me.

I agree to set personal boundaries for myself and others.

This is a form of respect.

I agree to do one thing each day to move me forward toward what I want.

I agree to thank my body for all the amazing things it does for me.

I agree to acknowledge that real women aren't perfect and perfect women are not real.

I agree to acknowledge that health comes in all shapes and sizes.

I agree to pursue my passions or learn more about them.

I agree to make healing my relationship with myself and food the priority.

I agree to turn to use new ways to manage my emotional state.

I agree to give myself permission to feel my feelings.

I agree to ask for help when I need it.

I agree to forgive myself and others for any perceived wrongdoings.

I agree to respect my body and honour its needs.

I agree to let go of anything necessary that no longer serves me.

Brenda J. Bentley

I agree to be grateful for everything, including challenges as I realize their importance in my self growth.

I agree to eat mindfully to increase satisfaction and pleasure in eating.

I agree to be more aware of my thoughts, feelings and behaviors.

I agree to STOP and take a moment to pause to be aware of myself and my surroundings.

I agree to nurture and love myself and others that are important to me.

Feel free to modify or add your own!

Chapter 17—A Transformation Story

"And the day came when the risk to remain tight in a bud was more painful than the risk it took to blossom."
~ Anaïs Nin

Everything contained in this book I have used personally on my own journey of transformation. I have walked on the same path you have. Life can thrust upon you situations and circumstances where you have no choice but to change or suffer being the same. The process of change happens when you decide it will and you commit yourself to learning the lessons along the way.

Our true self lies within our fears. You reclaim the energy and power of yourself when you venture into the territory you have willfully avoided. Every fear you confront and breakthrough expands your appreciation for who you are. If you feel afraid, it is a good indication that you are moving into a place where your personal power hides.

In my life I have broken through, and continue to breakthrough fear, and transform my belief in myself as I realize who I really am. This definition of myself is limitless, powerful, courageous, kind, loving, forgiving, helpful, compassionate, gentle, beautiful, open, expressive and authentic. Every day, I learn more and more about who I really am, and on this path of enlightenment, I know there is no destination. There is no place I am seeking to arrive.

There is nothing I need to do. There is nothing I need to have to complete me. I am complete. I am perfect just as I am. I had only temporarily forgotten this truth. Every experience I have been through served as a gentle reminder to wake up and be who I really am. It taught me to be me—THE WHOLE ME.

At the time of writing this, I am sitting on my sofa, in my living room on a Wednesday afternoon. I find myself wondering what

I am going to write. My publisher has asked me to change some of the contents of this chapter for legal reasons. I really had not been aware at time of submission that by writing about my past experiences, I was putting myself in a potential legal battle with the people that I claimed to be involved. So, here I sit, wondering what words will come.

I have spent many hours considering what words would come to explain to you the experiences I have had and how I have gone from being the person I was to the person I am today. I thought I could at first give you snapshots of my experiences, in a factual way to show you that I been through some awful and devastating abuse and come through it healthy, happy and self actualized.

The whole process of this book has been in itself transformational. The truth is, I needed to write this book to grow as the ruminants of those experiences still come up from time to time. This is an opportunity to re-write this chapter with even more balance and empowerment than I had before. The very act of challenging me to reconsider what voice I was using in writing this has transformed me.

When you begin the process of transformation, you soon begin to realize you never stop it. You are constantly evolving to a higher, truer expression of yourself. What an amazing thing that is to know, such a healing thought that everything changes and the process is constant and inevitable. It's only when you resist the process of change that you get yourself stuck.

With each chapter of this book you have been given the tools I have used to transform my own life from someone who felt depressed, fat, unlovable, unwanted, diseased, disempowered and dying to the person I am today.

My story of my past is only a series of experiences which have led me to become a person who can help other people transform themselves. I am certain, that if I had not had these experiences I would not have done so. It is true I used to regret that I had these experiences saying to myself "Only if I had this or that, my life would have been better." This regret kept me where I was, unable to accept myself or my experiences for many, many years.

There has been abuse in my past. I have been sexually abused, physically abused, emotionally and mentally abused. I have been abandoned and neglected. I was bullied in school and felt isolated and alone as I was moved around from place to place and attended over thirty schools before I left school at age 15. The lack of stability and uncertainty I felt made me independent but naive. When you have no choice but to be the new kid on the block you develop the ability to adapt and adapt fast. Call it a survival skill and for many years well into my adult life, I was in survival mode. When we are in survival mode, we rarely think outside of what we need to be happy or healthy individuals functioning in society. It's not a high priority to reach out and help others as we can barely help ourselves. You may be familiar with Abraham Maslow's Hierarchy of Needs:

1. Basic Biological and Physiological needs—food, drink, shelter, warmth, sleep, etc.

2. Safety needs—protection from elements, security, order, law, limits, stability, etc.

3. Belongingness and Love needs—work group, family, affection, relationships, etc.

4. Esteem needs—self-esteem, achievement, responsibility, etc.

5. Self-Actualization needs—realizing personal potential, self-fulfilment, seeking personal growth and peak experiences.

In order to move up to being a self-actualized individual, all the lower number levels needs must first be met. I certainly can say that in my own personal experience, my growth has only occurred after I have moved past survival mode into having my belonging / love / esteem needs met.

The result of being in survival mode meant that I had very little self esteem or self worth. I actually felt I had no value at all. I wasn't treated as someone who had self worth, I was abused, criticized and left to my own devices and this is the way I saw the world. I cannot pinpoint at which exact moment I made the decision that I had no value, but at a very young age, I remember feeling ugly, that I was no good and that my body was wrong.

As I grew into a teenager, the feelings became more profound as I compared myself and become very self conscious. I would cover up my perceived flaws (my freckles) with tons of make-up. I found myself in the company of other people who either bullied me or reinforced what I believed about myself. I wanted desperately to fit in and wanted to be accepted. This meant I often found myself in compromising situations which rarely ended in a favourable way.

Things didn't improve as experience after experience reinforced this limiting belief I held about myself, other people and the world. I turned to drugs and alcohol to help ease the pain and fill the void I felt inside.

All of this accumulated to a point in my life I was so desperately unhappy, I thought the world would be better off without me in it. I was tipping the scales at over 280 pounds and I felt my body was slowly dying from the inside out. It was about this time I was diagnosed with Hypo Thyroid Disease. My body was actually shutting down very, very slowly. I had given up all hope, and day after day repeated the same dithering irresolution of this meaningless existence of the half-lived life.

I think it was at my darkest moments when I had the biggest breakthroughs. It was as if in the desperation of giving up entirely something bigger than myself flicked a switch helping me to wake up from this sleepwalking state to the realization that I didn't want to live or die like this. I wanted to live. I wanted to be happy.

From that point, I began my transformation. I began with the decision to no longer stay the way I was. It was that simple. From that point I have exposed every lie, every hurt, every wound, every pain, every heartbreak, every fear I felt and shed these like a snake sheds its skin. Life seemed to thrust me into situations (and it still does) that reveal deeper levels of insecurities and limiting beliefs that I was, at that current level of consciousness, able to be aware of.

I went straight into my pain and I worked to let it all go.

I released the pain and the fear. I challenged my limiting beliefs and practised a new way of thinking about myself. I learned to love and accept myself just as I am. I forgave everyone who ever hurt me. I forgave myself for hurting me and for hurting others. I renewed myself through the process I have shared with you. I continue this process every day. I know there are even more gifts awaiting me being open to seeing them. I know I am safe in all that I do. No matter how painful life is, how desperate I can feel at times, I know on the other side of this, is a truer expression of who I really am.

To be whole and fulfilled, you must be willing to accept everything you are. EVERYTHING. The good, the bad, the ugly, the painful, the hurt, the pain, the mistakes, the fears . . . I admit that I am still in the process of accepting everything about myself that I have dismissed, disowned and repressed. These parts of you that you try to hide from others. We go into the world wanting everyone to see only the best of us. We hide our insecurities and our fears and work hard to suppress them, until one day they come up and bite us on the backside!

In order to realize the truest expression of yourself, you will need to fully integrate all these parts of you so you can create a connection with this part and realize that it is giving you the opportunity to be whole again. Everything you fear is only your strength exiled. Trust yourself to know you can do this. If you don't believe in yourself, then remember that I believe in you.

Resources

Download free self hypnosis and guided meditations plus additional resources to support your transformation. You may also want to purchase the Eat, Guilt, Repent, Repeat Companion Workbook and Audio Toolkit from www.eatguiltrepentrepeat.com

References

Mann, T. (2007). Medicare's search for effective obesity treatments: Diets are not the answer. American Psychologist, 62(3): 220-233.

Stryer, Lubert (2002). Biochemistry: Metabolism, Basic Concepts and Design, 14.

Keys, A.; Bro_ek, J.; Henschel, A.; Mickelsen, O.; Taylor,

H. L. (1950). the Biology of Human Starvation. Oxford,

England: Univ. of Minnesota Press. xxxii 1385.

Rumsey, N.; Harcourt, D. (2003). Body image and disfigurement: issues and interventions. Centre for Appearance Research, University of the West of England, 87.

Mustillo, A., Hendrix, K. and Schafer, M. (2012). Trajectories of Body Mass and Self-Concept in Black and White Girls: The Lingering Effects of Stigma. Journal of Health and Social Behavior; vol. 53, 1: 2-16.

James, W. (1890). The Principles of Psychology. Chapter IV, Habit. Ch. 4, 122-123.

Moseley, B., et al. (2002). Controlled Trial of Arthroscopic Surgery for Osteoarthritis of the Knee. The New England Journal of Medicine, 347:81-88.

Davidson, R., Kabat-Zinn, J., et al. (2003). Alterations in brain and immune function produced by mindfulness meditation. Psychosomatic Medicine, 65, 564-570.

Seligman, M. (1998). Learned Optimism: How to Change Your Mind and Your Life.

Emmons, R., McCullough, M. (2003). Counting blessings versus burdens: An experimental investigation of gratitude and subjective well-being in daily life. Journal of Personality and Social Psychology, Vol. 84, No. 2, 377-389.

Tribole, E., Resch, E. (2003). 10 Principles of Intuitive Eating. Intuitive Eating, 20-29.

Guiliana, M. (2005). French Women Don't Get Fat.

Printed in Great Britain
by Amazon